The Mediterranean Salad Bible

Healthy and Vibrant Savory Dishes with Vegetables and Fresh Produce

By
Delia Bell

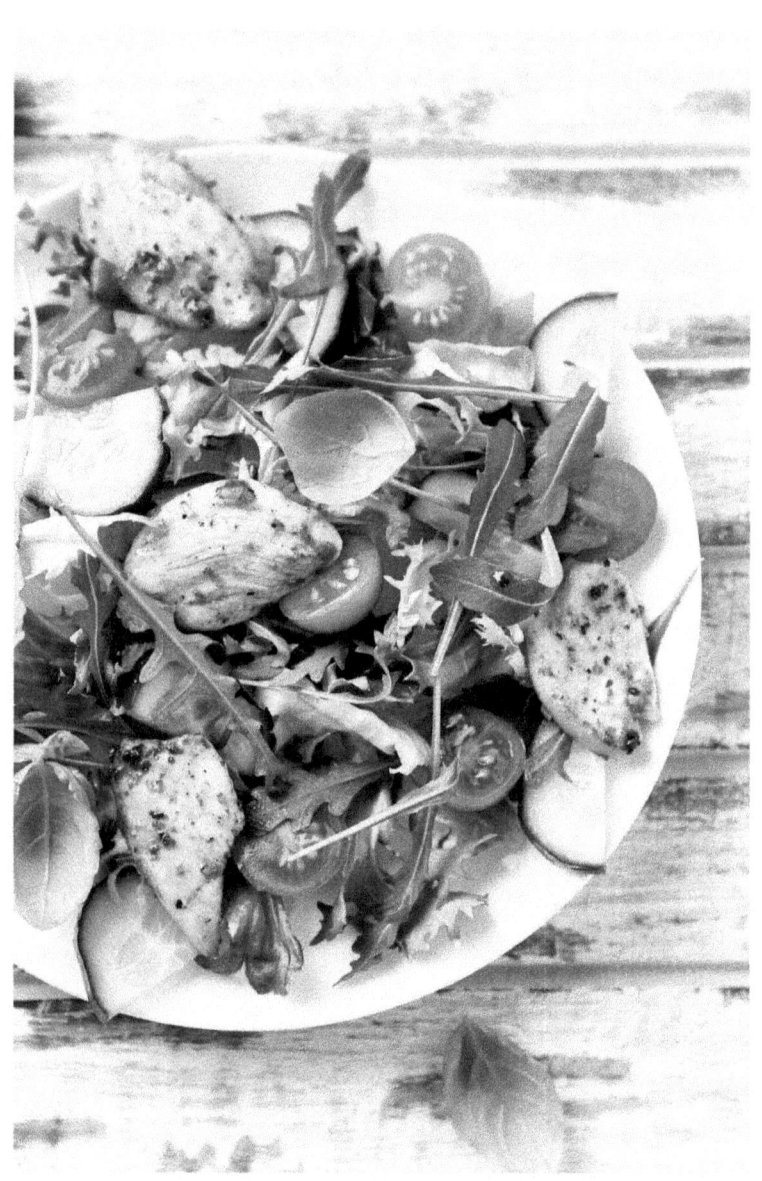

© Copyright 2021 by Delia Bell - All rights reserved. The following Book is reproduced below with the goal of providing information that is as accurate and reliable as possible. Regardless, purchasing this Book can be seen as consent to the fact that both the publisher and the author of this book are in no way experts on the topics discussed within and that any recommendations or suggestions that are made herein are for entertainment purposes only. Professionals should be consulted as needed prior to undertaking any of the action endorsed herein.

This declaration is deemed fair and valid by both the American Bar Association and the Committee of Publishers Association and is legally binding throughout the United States.

Furthermore, the transmission, duplication, or reproduction of any of the following work including specific information will be considered an illegal act irrespective of if it is done electronically or in print. This extends to creating a secondary or tertiary copy of the work or a recorded copy and is only allowed with the express written consent from the Publisher. All additional rights reserved.

The information in the following pages is broadly considered a truthful and accurate account of facts and as such, any inattention, use, or misuse of the information in question by the reader will render any resulting actions solely under their purview. There are no scenarios in which the publisher or the original author of this work can be in any fashion deemed liable for any hardship or damages that may befall them after undertaking information described herein.

Additionally, the information in the following pages is intended only for informational purposes and should thus be thought of as universal. As befitting its nature, it is presented without assurance regarding its prolonged validity or interim quality. Trademarks that are mentioned are done without written consent and can in no way be considered an endorsement from the trademark holder.

Table of Contents

INTRODUCTION   7
- What is the Mediterranean Diet?   7
- Quinoa Salad   13
- Couscous And Toasted Almonds   14
- Spanish Tomato Salad   16
- Chickpeas And Beets Mix   17
- Roasted Bell Pepper Salad With Anchovy Dressing   19
- Warm Shrimp And Arugula Salad   20
- Cheesy Tomato Salad   21
- Garlic Cucumber Mix   22
- Cucumber Salad Japanese Style   24
- Cheesy Keto Zucchini Soup   25
- Grilled Salmon Summer Salad   27
- Dill Beets Salad   29
- Green Couscous With Broad Beans, Pistachio, And Dill   31
- Bell Peppers Salad   33
- Thyme Corn And Cheese Mix   35
- Garden Salad With Oranges And Olives   36
- Smoked Salmon Lentil Salad   39
- Salmon & Arugula Salad   40
- Keto Bbq Chicken Pizza Soup   43
- Mediterranean Garden Salad   45
- Buttery Millet   48
- Delicata Squash Soup   49
- Parsley Couscous And Cherries Salad   52
- Mint Quinoa   53
- Spicy Halibut Tomato Soup   56
- Beans With Pancetta, Sage, And Vinegar   58

Mediterranean-style Vegetable Stew	61
Cheesy Potatoes	63
Greek Beets	65
Snow Peas Salad	66
Beans And Rice	68
Parsley Tomato Mix	69
Lemon Chili Cucumbers	71
Tuna-dijon Salad	72
Grilled Chicken Salad	75
Chili Cabbage And Coconut	77
Spinach And Cranberry Salad	79
Dill Cucumber Salad	81
Nutty, Curry-citrus Garden Salad	83
Mouthwatering Steakhouse Salad	84
Green Beans With Pomegranate Dressing	87
Cauliflower And Thyme Soup	89
Turkey Maghiritsa	90
Quinoa And Greens Salad	92
Mushroom Spinach Soup	94
Spicy Herb Potatoes (batata Harra)	96
Orange Couscous	99
Walnuts Cucumber Mix	100
Red Beet Spinach Salad	102
Broccoli Spaghetti	103
Leeks Sauté	105
Whole-wheat Soft Dinner Dough And Rolls	106
Peppers And Lentils Salad	109

INTRODUCTION

What is the Mediterranean Diet?

The Mediterranean diet is based on the diets of traditional eating habits from the 1960s of people from countries that surround the Mediterranean Sea, such as Greece, Italy, and Spain, and it encourages the consumption of fresh, seasonal, and local foods. The Mediterranean diet has become popular because individuals show low rates of heart disease, chronic disease, and obesity. The Mediterranean diet profile focuses on whole grains, good fats (fish, olive oil, nuts etc.), vegetables, fruits, fish, and very low consumption of any non-fish meat. Along with food, the Mediterranean diet emphasizes the need to spend time eating with family and physical activity. The Mediterranean diet is not a single prescribed diet, but rather a general food-based eating pattern, which is marked by local and cultural differences throughout the Mediterranean region.

The diet is generally characterized by a high intake of plant-based foods (e.g. fresh fruit and vegetables, nuts, and cereals) and olive oil, a moderate intake of fish and poultry, and low intakes of dairy products (mostly yoghurt and cheese), red and processed meats, and sweets. Wine is typically consumed in moderation and, normally, with a meal. A strong focus is placed on social and cultural aspects, such as communal mealtimes, resting after eating, and regular physical activity. Nowadays, however, the diet is no longer followed as widely as it was 30-50 years ago, as the diets of people living in these regions are becoming more 'Westernized' and higher in energy dense foods.

Benefits
The Mediterranean diet is not a weight loss, but increasing fiber intake and cutting out red meat, animal fats, and processed food may lead to weight loss. People who follow the diet may also have a lower risk of various diseases.

Heart health
In the 1950s, an American scientist, found that people living in the poorer areas of southern Italy had a lower risk of heart disease and death than those in wealthier parts of New York. Dr. Keys attributed this to diet. Since then, many studies have indicated that following a Mediterranean diet can help the body maintain healthy cholesterol levels and reduce the risk of high blood pressure and cardiovascular disease. The overall pattern of the Mediterranean diet is similar to their own dietary recommendations. A high proportion of calories on the diet come from fat, which can increase the risk of obesity. However, they also note that this fat is mainly unsaturated, which makes it a more healthful option than that from the typical American diet.

Protection from disease
The Mediterranean diet focuses on plant-based foods, and these are good sources of antioxidants.

The Mediterranean diet might offer protection from various cancers, and especially colorectal cancer. The reduction in risk may stem from the high intake of fruits, vegetables, and whole grains. By sticking to Mediterranean meals, people's levels of blood glucose and fats had decreased. During this time, there was also a lower incidence of stroke.

Diabetes
The Mediterranean diet may help prevent type 2 diabetes and improve markers of diabetes in people who already have the condition. Various other studies have concluded that following the Mediterranean diet can reduce the risk of type 2 diabetes and cardiovascular disease, which often occur together.

Food to eat
There is no single definition of the Mediterranean diet, but one group of scientists used the following as their 2015 basis of research.

Vegetables: Include 3 to 9 servings a day.

Fresh fruit: Up to 2 servings a day.

Cereals: Mostly whole grain from 1 to 13 servings a day.

Oil: Up to 8 servings of extra virgin (cold pressed) olive oil a day.

Fat — mostly unsaturated — made up 37% of the total calories. Unsaturated fat comes from plant sources, such as olives and avocado. The Mediterranean diet also provided 33 grams (g) of fiber a day. The baseline diet for this study provided around

2,200 calories a day. Typical ingredients. Here are some examples of ingredients that people often include in the Mediterranean diet.

Vegetables: Tomatoes, peppers, onions, eggplant, zucchini, cucumber, leafy green vegetables, plus others.
Fruits: Melon, apples, apricots, peaches, oranges, and lemons, and so on.
Legumes: Beans, lentils, and chickpeas.
Nuts and seeds: Almonds, walnuts, sunflower seeds, and cashews.
Unsaturated fat: Olive oil, sunflower oil, olives, and avocados.
Dairy products: Cheese and yogurt are the main dairy foods.
Cereals: These are mostly whole grain and include wheat and rice with bread accompanying many meals.
Fish: Sardines and other oily fish, as well as oysters and other shellfish. Poultry: Chicken or turkey.
Eggs: Chicken, quail, and duck eggs.
Drinks: A person can drink red wine in moderation.

The Mediterranean diet does not include strong liquor or carbonated and sweetened drinks. According to one definition, the diet limits red meat and sweets to less than 2 servings per week.

Food to avoid
Here's a list of foods you should generally limit while eating Mediterranean-style meals. Heavily processed foods. Let's be real: Many, many foods are processed to some degree. A can of beans has been processed, in the sense that the beans have been cooked before being canned. Olive oil has been processed, because olives have been turned into oil. But when we talk about limiting processed foods, this really means avoiding things like frozen meals with tons of sodium. You should also limit soda, desserts and candy. As the adage goes, if the ingredient list includes items that your great-grandparents wouldn't recognize as food, it's probably processed. If you're buying a packaged food that's as close to its whole-food form as possible — such as frozen fruit or veggies with nothing added — you're good to go.

Processed red meat
On the Mediterranean diet, you should minimize your intake of red meat, such as steak. What about processed red meat, such as hot dogs and bacon? You should avoid these foods or limit them as much as possible. A study published in BMJ found that regularly eating red meat, especially processed varieties, was associated with a higher risk of death. Butter. Here's another food that should be limited on the Mediterranean diet. Use olive oil instead, which has many heart health benefits and contains less saturated fat than butter. According to the USDA National Nutrient Database, butter has 7 grams of saturated fat per tablespoon, while olive oil has about 2 grams.

Refined grains

The Mediterranean diet is centered around whole grains, such as farro, millet, couscous and brown rice. With this eating style, you'll generally want to limit your intake of refined grains such as white pasta and white bread.

Alcohol

When you're following the Mediterranean diet, red wine should be your chosen alcoholic drink. This is because red wine offers health benefits, particularly for the heart. But it's important to limit intake of any type of alcohol to up to one drink per day for women, as well as men older than 65, and up to two drinks daily for men age 65 and younger. The amount that counts as a drink is 5 ounces of wine, 12 ounces of beer or 1.5 ounces of 80-proof liquor.

Quinoa Salad

Servings: 2 Cups

Cooking Time: 20 Minutes

Ingredients:
- 2 cups red quinoa
- 4 cups water
- 1 (15-oz.) can chickpeas, drained
- 1 medium red onion, chopped (1/2 cup)
- 3 TB. fresh mint leaves, finely chopped
- 1/4 cup extra-virgin olive oil
- 3 TB. fresh lemon juice
- 1/2 tsp. salt
- 1/2 tsp. fresh ground black pepper

Directions:

1. In a medium saucepan over medium-high heat, bring red quinoa and water to a boil. Cover, reduce heat to low, and cook for 20 minutes or until water is absorbed and quinoa is tender. Let cool.
2. In a large bowl, add quinoa, chickpeas, red onion, and mint.
3. In a small bowl, whisk together extra-virgin olive oil, lemon juice, salt, and black pepper.
4. Pour dressing over quinoa mixture, and stir well to combine.
5. Serve immediately, or refrigerate and enjoy for up to 2 or 3 days.

Couscous And Toasted Almonds

Servings: 4
Cooking Time: 10 Minutes

Ingredients:
- 1 cup (about 200 g) whole-grain couscous
- 400 ml boiling water
- 1 tablespoon extra-virgin olive oil
- 1/2 red onion, chopped
- 1/2 teaspoon ground ginger,
- 1/2 teaspoon ground cinnamon and
- 1/2 teaspoon ground coriander
- 2 tablespoons blanched almonds, toasted, and chopped

Directions:
1. Preheat the oven to 110C.
2. In a casserole, toss the couscous with the olive oil, onion, spices, salt and pepper. Stir in the boiling water, cover, and bake for 10 minutes. Fluff using a fork. Scatter the nuts over the top and then serve. Pair with harira.

Nutrition Info:Per Serving:261.23 cal,8 g total fat (1 g sat. fat), 37 g carb, 7 g protein, 1 g sugar, and 6.85 mg sodium.

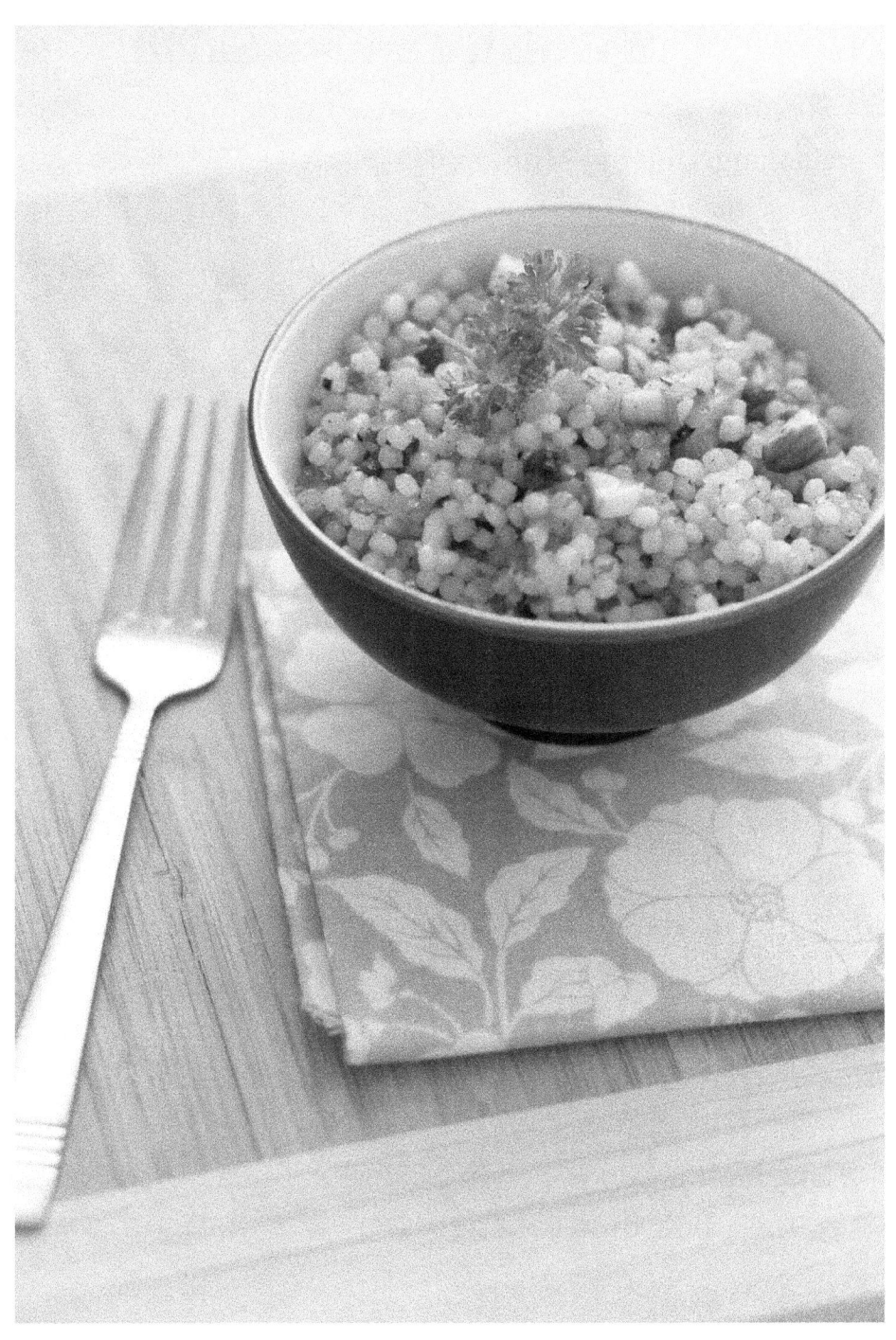

Spanish Tomato Salad

Servings: 4
Cooking Time: 15 Minutes

Ingredients:
- 1 pound tomatoes, cubed
- 2 cucumbers, cubed
- 2 garlic cloves, chopped
- 1 red onion, sliced
- 2 anchovy fillets
- 1 tablespoon balsamic vinegar
- 1 pinch chili powder
- Salt and pepper to taste

Directions:
1. Combine the tomatoes, cucumbers, garlic and red onion in a bowl.
2. In a mortar, mix the anchovy fillets, vinegar, chili powder, salt and pepper.
3. Drizzle the mixture over the salad and mix well.
4. Serve the salad fresh.

Nutrition Info: Per Serving:Calories: 61 Fat: 0.6g Protein: 3.0g Carbohydrates: 13.0g

Chickpeas And Beets Mix

Servings: 4

Cooking Time: 25 Minutes

Ingredients:
- 3 tablespoons capers, drained and chopped
- Juice of 1 lemon
- Zest of 1 lemon, grated
- 1 red onion, chopped
- 3 tablespoons olive oil
- 14 ounces canned chickpeas, drained
- 8 ounces beets, peeled and cubed
- 1 tablespoon parsley, chopped
- Salt and pepper to the taste

Directions:

1. Heat up a pan with the oil over medium heat, add the onion, lemon zest, lemon juice and the capers and sauté fro 5 minutes.
2. Add the rest of the ingredients, stir and cook over medium-low heat for 20 minutes more.
3. Divide the mix between plates and serve as a side dish.

Nutrition Info: calories 199, fat 4.5, fiber 2.3, carbs 6.5, protein 3.3

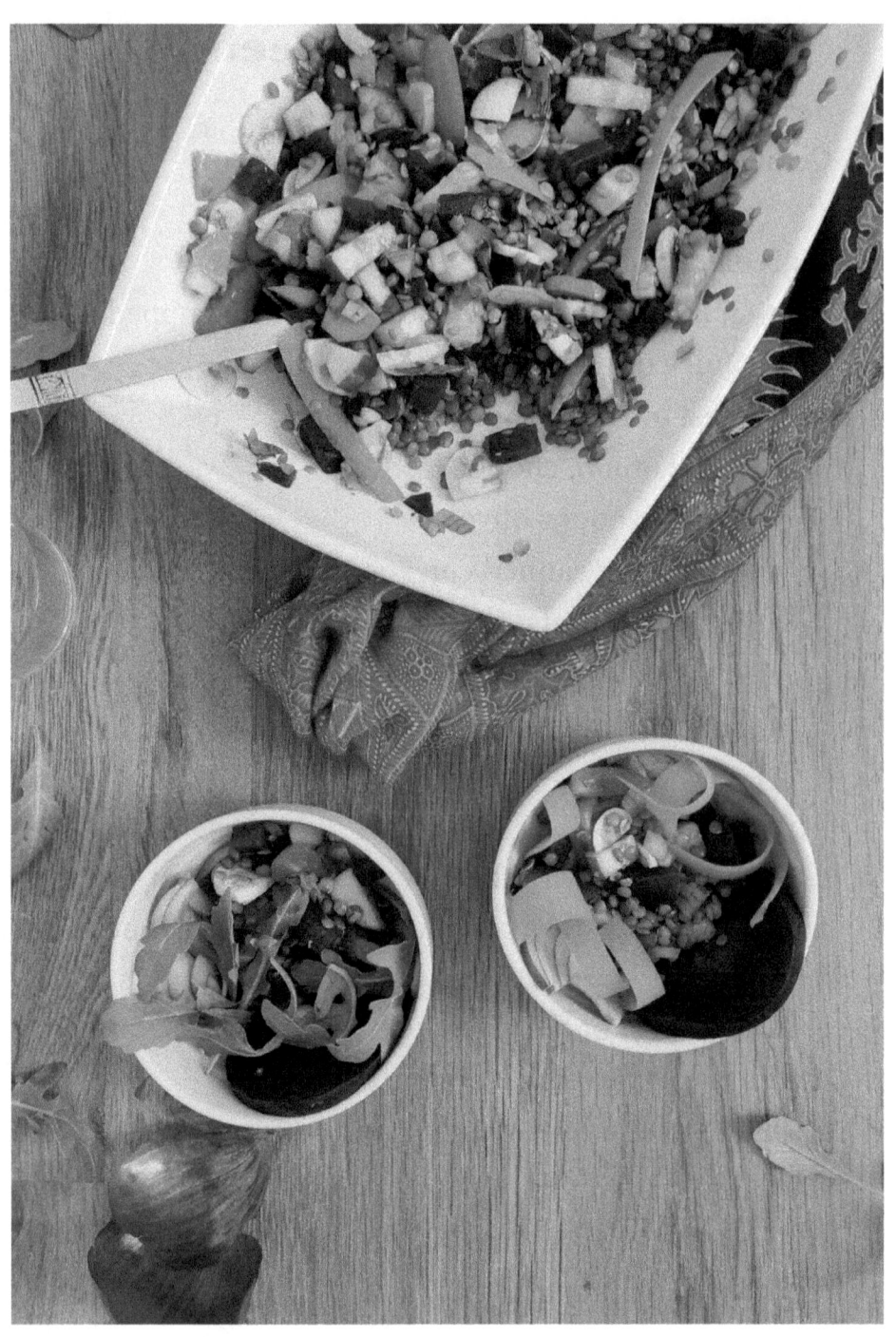

Roasted Bell Pepper Salad With Anchovy Dressing

Servings: 4
Cooking Time: 20 Minutes

Ingredients:
- 8 roasted red bell peppers, sliced
- 2 tablespoons pine nuts
- 1 cup cherry tomatoes, halved
- 2 tablespoons chopped parsley
- 4 anchovy fillets
- 1 lemon, juiced
- 1 garlic clove
- 1 tablespoon extra-virgin olive oil
- Salt and pepper to taste

Directions:
1. Combine the anchovy fillets, lemon juice, garlic and olive oil in a mortar and mix them well.
2. Mix the rest of the ingredients in a salad bowl then drizzle in the dressing.
3. Serve the salad as fresh as possible.

Nutrition Info: Per Serving: Calories: 81 Fat: 7.0g Protein: 2.4g Carbohydrates: 4.0g

Warm Shrimp And Arugula Salad

Servings: 4

Cooking Time: 20 Minutes

Ingredients:
- 2 tablespoons extra virgin olive oil
- 2 garlic cloves, minced
- 1 red pepper, sliced
- 1 pound fresh shrimps, peeled and deveined
- 1 orange, juiced
- Salt and pepper to taste
- 3 cups arugula

Directions:

1. Heat the oil in a frying pan and stir in the garlic and red pepper. Cook for 1 minute then add the shrimps.
2. Cook for 5 minutes then add the orange juice and cook for another 5 more minutes.
3. When done, spoon the shrimps and the sauce over the arugula.
4. Serve the salad fresh.

Nutrition Info: Per Serving:Calories:232 Fat:9.2g Protein:27.0g Carbohydrates:10.0g

Cheesy Tomato Salad

Servings: 4

Cooking Time: 0 Minutes

Ingredients:
- 2 pounds tomatoes, sliced
- 1 red onion, chopped
- Sea salt and black pepper to the taste
- 4 ounces feta cheese, crumbled
- 2 tablespoons mint, chopped
- A drizzle of olive oil

Directions:

1. In a salad bowl, mix the tomatoes with the onion and the rest of the ingredients, toss and serve as a side salad.

Nutrition Info: calories 190, fat 4.5, fiber 3.4, carbs 8.7, protein 3.3

Garlic Cucumber Mix

Servings: 4
Cooking Time: 0 Minutes

Ingredients:
- 2 cucumbers, sliced
- 2 spring onions, chopped
- 2 tablespoons olive oil
- 3 garlic cloves, grated
- 1 tablespoon thyme, chopped
- Salt and black pepper to the taste
- 3 and ½ ounces goat cheese, crumbled

Directions:
1. In a salad bowl, mix the cucumbers with the onions and the rest of the ingredients, toss and serve after keeping it in the fridge for 15 minutes.

Nutrition Info: calories 140, fat 5.4, fiber 4.3, carbs 6.5, protein 4.8

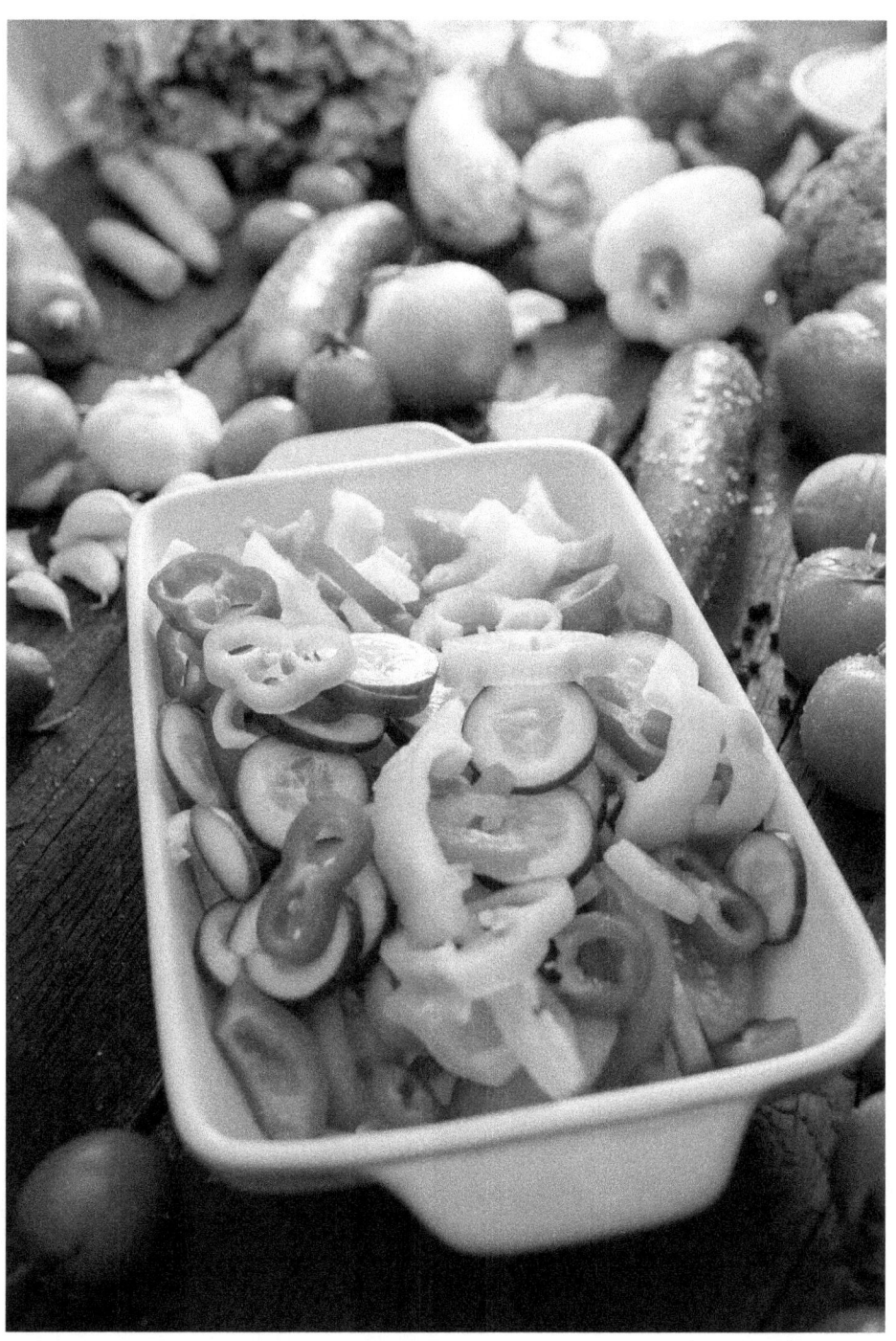

Cucumber Salad Japanese Style

Servings: 5

Cooking Time: 0 Minutes

Ingredients:
- 1 ½ tsp minced fresh ginger root
- 1 tsp salt
- 1/3 cup rice vinegar
- 2 large cucumbers, ribbon cut
- 4 tsp white sugar

Directions:
1. Mix well ginger, salt, sugar and vinegar in a small bowl.
2. Add ribbon cut cucumbers and mix well.
3. Let stand for at least one hour in the ref before serving.

Nutrition Info: Calories per Serving: 29; Fat: .2g; Protein: .7g; Carbs: 6.1g

Cheesy Keto Zucchini Soup

Servings: 2

Cooking Time: 20 Minutes

Ingredients:
- ½ medium onion, peeled and chopped
- 1 cup bone broth
- 1 tablespoon coconut oil
- 1½ zucchinis, cut into chunks
- ½ tablespoon nutritional yeast
- Dash of black pepper
- ½ tablespoon parsley, chopped, for garnish
- ½ tablespoon coconut cream, for garnish

Directions:
1. Melt the coconut oil in a large pan over medium heat and add onions.
2. Sauté for about 3 minutes and add zucchinis and bone broth.
3. Reduce the heat to simmer for about 15 minutes and cover the pan.
4. Add nutritional yeast and transfer to an immersion blender.
5. Blend until smooth and season with black pepper.
6. Top with coconut cream and parsley to serve.

Nutrition Info: Calories: 154 Carbs: 8.9g Fats: 8.1g Proteins: 13.4g Sodium: 93mg Sugar: 3.9g

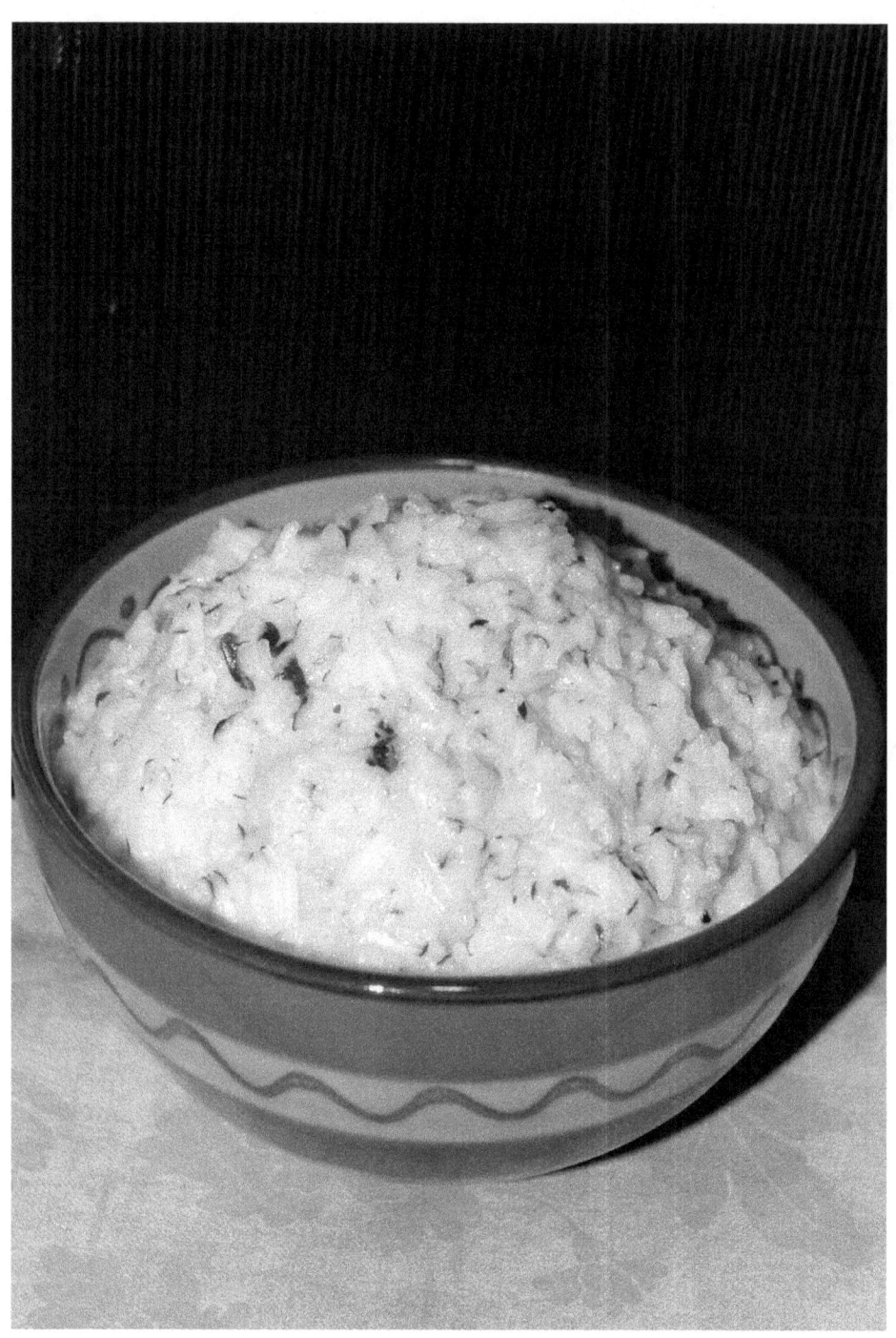

Grilled Salmon Summer Salad

Servings: 4

Cooking Time: 30 Minutes

Ingredients:
- Salmon fillets - 2
- Salt and pepper - to taste
- Vegetable stock - 2 cups
- Bulgur - 1 2 cup
- Cherry tomatoes - 1 cup, halved
- Sweet corn - 1 2 cup
- Lemon - 1, juiced
- Green olives - 1 2 cup, sliced
- Cucumber - 1, cubed
- Green onion - 1, chopped
- Red pepper - 1, chopped
- Red bell pepper - 1, cored and diced

Directions:

1. Heat a grill pan on medium and then place salmon on, seasoning with salt and pepper. Grill both sides of salmon until brown and set aside.

2. Heat stock in sauce pan until hot and then add in bulgur and cook until liquid is completely soaked into bulgur.

3. Mix salmon, bulgur and all other Ingredients in a salad bowl and again add salt and pepper, if desired, to suit your taste.

4. Serve salad as soon as completed.

Dill Beets Salad

Servings: 6

Cooking Time: 0 Minutes

Ingredients:
- 2 pounds beets, cooked, peeled and cubed
- 2 tablespoons olive oil
- 1 tablespoon lemon juice
- 2 tablespoons balsamic vinegar
- 1 cup feta cheese, crumbled
- 3 small garlic cloves, minced
- 4 green onions, chopped
- 5 tablespoons parsley, chopped
- Salt and black pepper to the taste

Directions:

1. In a bowl, mix the beets with the oil, lemon juice and the rest of the ingredients, toss and serve as a side dish.

Nutrition Info: calories 268, fat 15.5, fiber 5.1, carbs 25.7, protein 9.6

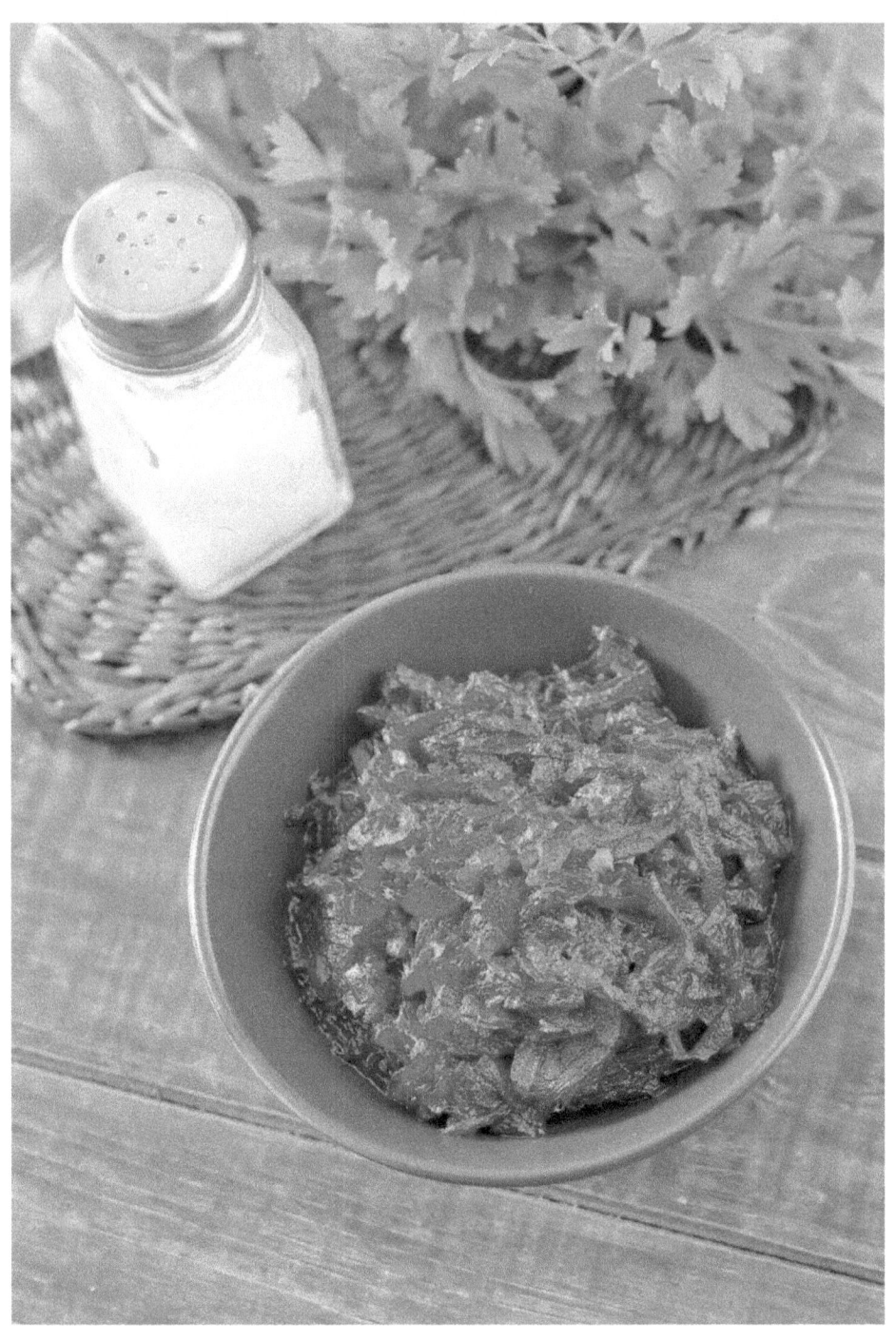

Green Couscous With Broad Beans, Pistachio, And Dill

Servings: 4

Cooking Time: 8 Minutes

Ingredients:

- 200 g fresh or frozen broad beans, podded
- 2 teaspoons ground ginger
- 2 tablespoons spring onion, thinly sliced
- 2 tablespoons pistachio kernels, roughly chopped
- 2 tablespoons lemon juice, and wedges to serve
- Dill, chopped - 1/4 cup
- Olive oil, extra-virgin - 1/4 cup (about 60 ml)
- 1/2 onion, thinly sliced
- Watercress, leaves picked - 1/2 bunch
- 1/2 avocado, chopped
- 1 green bell pepper, thinly sliced
- 1 garlic clove, crushed
- 1 cup (about 200 g) whole-grain couscous
- 1 1/2 cups boiling water

Directions:

1. In a heat-safe bowl, toss the couscous with the ginger and the onion. Stir in the boiling water, cover and let stand for 5 minutes.

2. Meanwhile, cook the beans for about 3 minutes in boiling salted water, drain, and refresh under running cold water; discard the outer skins.
3. With a fork, fluff the couscous. Add the beans, avocado, bell pepper, spring onion, and dill.
4. In a bowl, whisk the olive oil, lemon juice, and garlic; toss with the couscous. Scatter the pistacchio over the mix, serve with cress and the lemon wedges.

Nutrition Info:Per Serving:608 cal, 25.40 g total fat (4 g sat. fat), 51.50 g carb, 18.10 g protein, 45 mg sodium, and 11 g fiber.

Bell Peppers Salad

Servings: 6

Cooking Time: 0 Minutes

Ingredients:
- 2 green bell peppers, cut into thick strips
- 2 red bell peppers, cut into thick strips
- 2 tablespoons olive oil
- 1 garlic clove, minced
- ½ cup goat cheese, crumbled
- A pinch of salt and black pepper

Directions:

1. In a bowl, mix the bell peppers with the garlic and the other ingredients, toss and serve.

Nutrition Info: calories 193, fat 4.5, fiber 2, carbs 4.3, protein 3

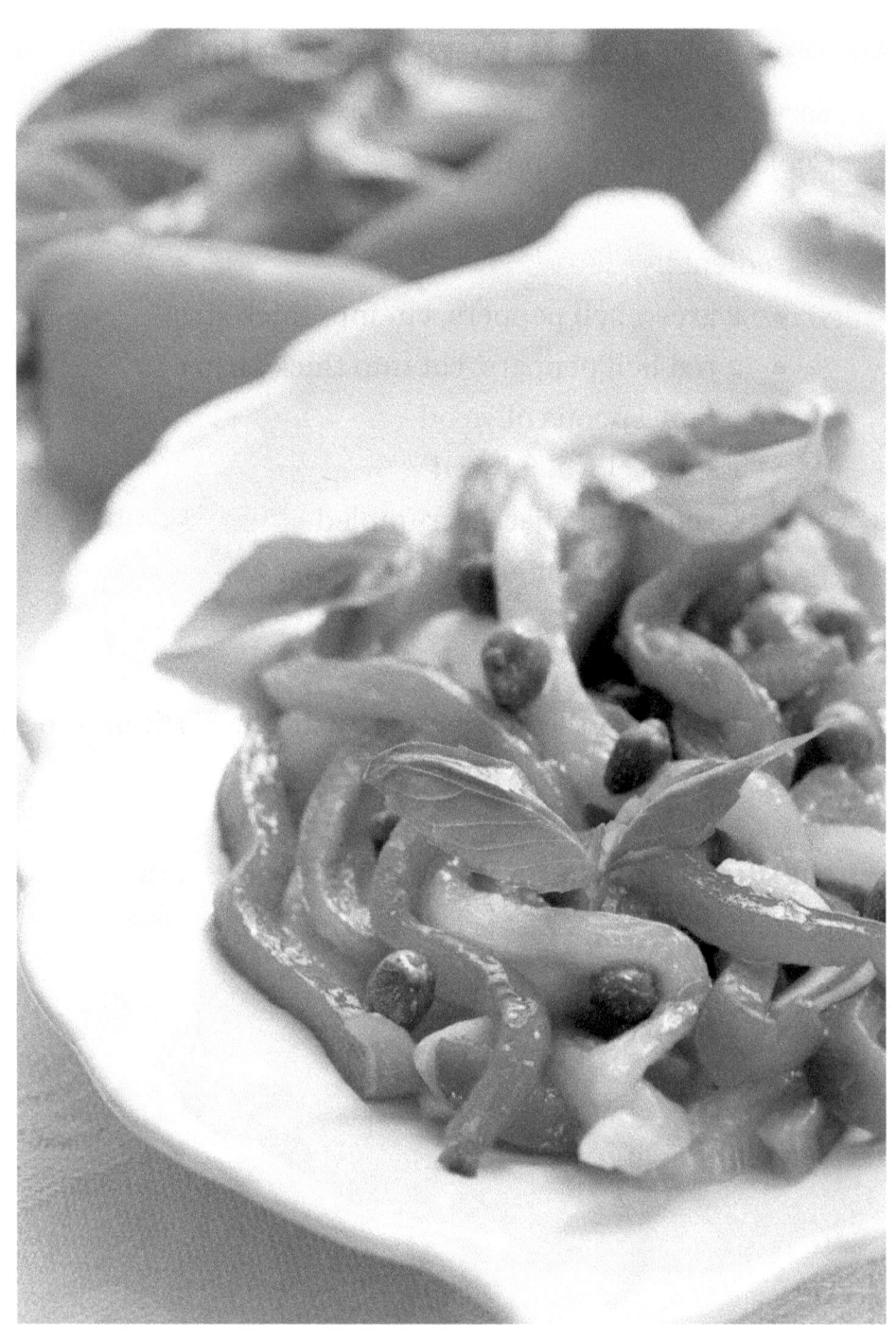

Thyme Corn And Cheese Mix

Servings: 4

Cooking Time: 0 Minutes

Ingredients:
- 1 tablespoon olive oil
- 1 teaspoon thyme, chopped
- 1 cup scallions, sliced
- 2 cups corn
- Salt and black pepper to the taste
- 2 tablespoons blue cheese, crumbled
- 1 tablespoon chives, chopped

Directions:

1. In a salad bowl, combine the corn with scallions, thyme and the rest of the ingredients, toss, divide between plates and serve.

Nutrition Info: calories 183, fat 5.5, fiber 7.5, carbs 14.5

Garden Salad With Oranges And Olives

Servings: 4
Cooking Time: 15 Minutes

Ingredients:
- ½ cup red wine vinegar
- 1 tbsp extra virgin olive oil
- 1 tbsp finely chopped celery
- 1 tbsp finely chopped red onion
- 16 large ripe black olives
- 2 garlic cloves
- 2 navel oranges, peeled and segmented
- 4 boneless, skinless chicken breasts, 4-oz each
- 4 garlic cloves, minced
- 8 cups leaf lettuce, washed and dried
- Cracked black pepper to taste

Directions:
1. Prepare the dressing by mixing pepper, celery, onion, olive oil, garlic and vinegar in a small bowl. Whisk well to combine.
2. Lightly grease grate and preheat grill to high.
3. Rub chicken with the garlic cloves and discard garlic.
4. Grill chicken for 5 minutes per side or until cooked through.

5. Remove from grill and let it stand for 5 minutes before cutting into ½- inch strips.

6. In 4 serving plates, evenly arrange two cups lettuce, ¼ of the sliced oranges and 4 olives per plate.

7. Top each plate with ¼ serving of grilled chicken, evenly drizzle with dressing, serve and enjoy.

Nutrition Info: Calories per serving: 259.8; Protein: 48.9g; Carbs: 12.9g; Fat: 1.4g

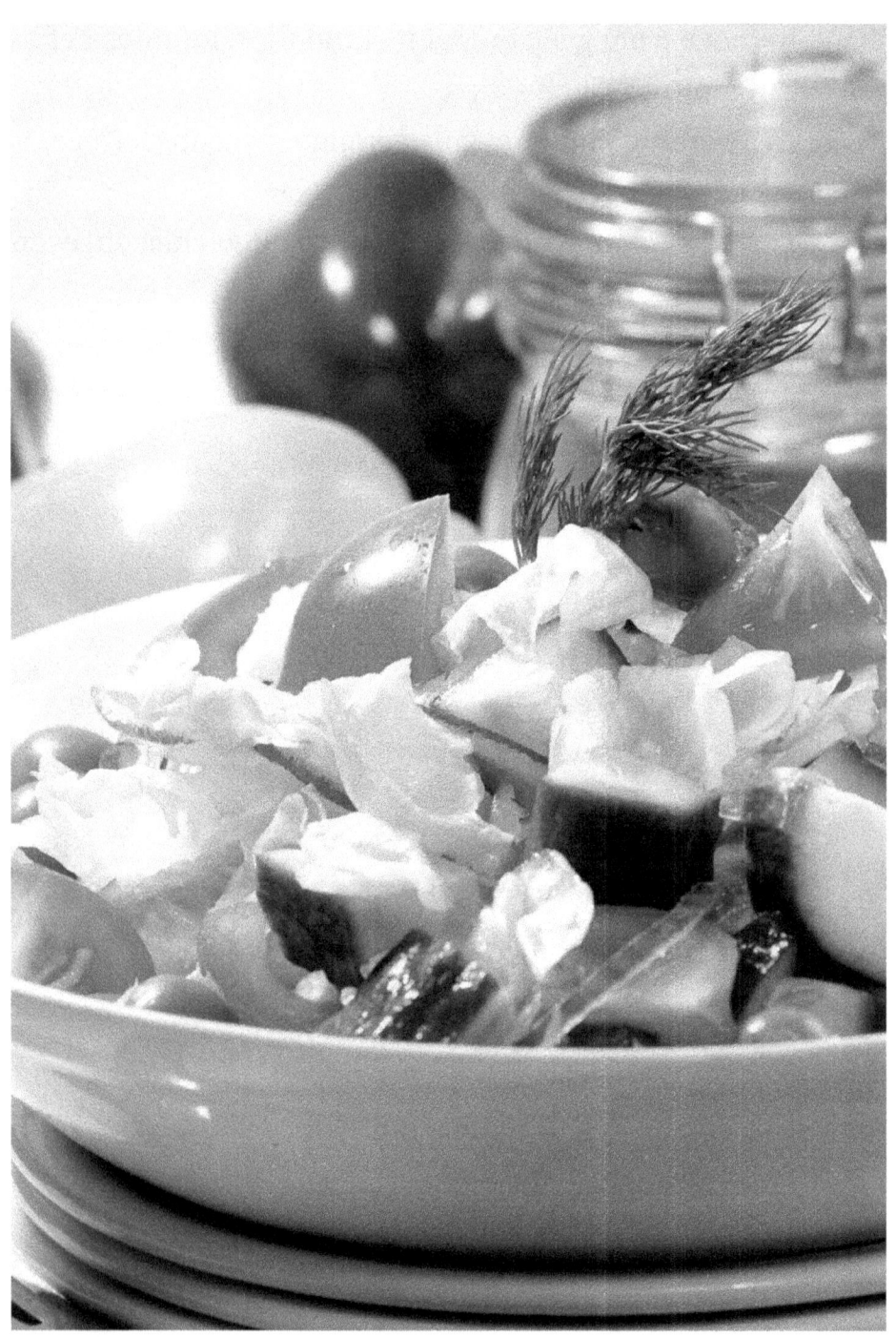

Smoked Salmon Lentil Salad

Servings: 4

Cooking Time: 25 Minutes

Ingredients:
- 1 cup green lentils, rinsed
- 2 cups vegetable stock
- ½ cup chopped parsley
- 2 tablespoons chopped cilantro
- 1 red pepper, chopped
- 1 red onion, chopped
- Salt and pepper to taste
- 4 oz. smoked salmon, shredded
- 1 lemon, juiced

Directions:

1. Combine the lentils and stock in a saucepan. Cook on low heat for 15-20 minutes or until all the liquid has been absorbed completely.
2. Transfer the lentils in a salad bowl and add the parsley, cilantro, red pepper and onion. Season with salt and pepper.
3. Add the smoked salmon and lemon juice and mix well.
4. Serve the salad fresh.

Nutrition Info: Per Serving:Calories:233 Fat:2.0g Protein:18.7g Carbohydrates:35.5g

Salmon & Arugula Salad

Servings: 2

Cooking Time: 12 Minutes

Ingredients:
- ¼ cup red onion, sliced thinly
- 1 ½ tbsp fresh lemon juice
- 1 ½ tbsp olive oil
- 1 tbsp extra-virgin olive oil
- 1 tbsp red-wine vinegar
- 2 center cut salmon fillets (6-oz each)
- 2/3 cup cherry tomatoes, halved
- 3 cups baby arugula leaves
- Pepper and salt to taste

Directions:

1. In a shallow bowl, mix pepper, salt, 1 ½ tbsp olive oil and lemon juice. Toss in salmon fillets and rub with the marinade. Allow to marinate for at least 15 minutes.
2. Grease a baking sheet and preheat oven to 350oF.
3. Bake marinated salmon fillet for 10 to 12 minutes or until flaky with skin side touching the baking sheet.
4. Meanwhile, in a salad bowl mix onion, tomatoes and arugula.

5. Season with pepper and salt. Drizzle with vinegar and oil. Toss to combine and serve right away with baked salmon on the side.

Nutrition Info: Calories per serving: 400; Protein: 36.6g; Carbs: 5.8g; Fat: 25.6g

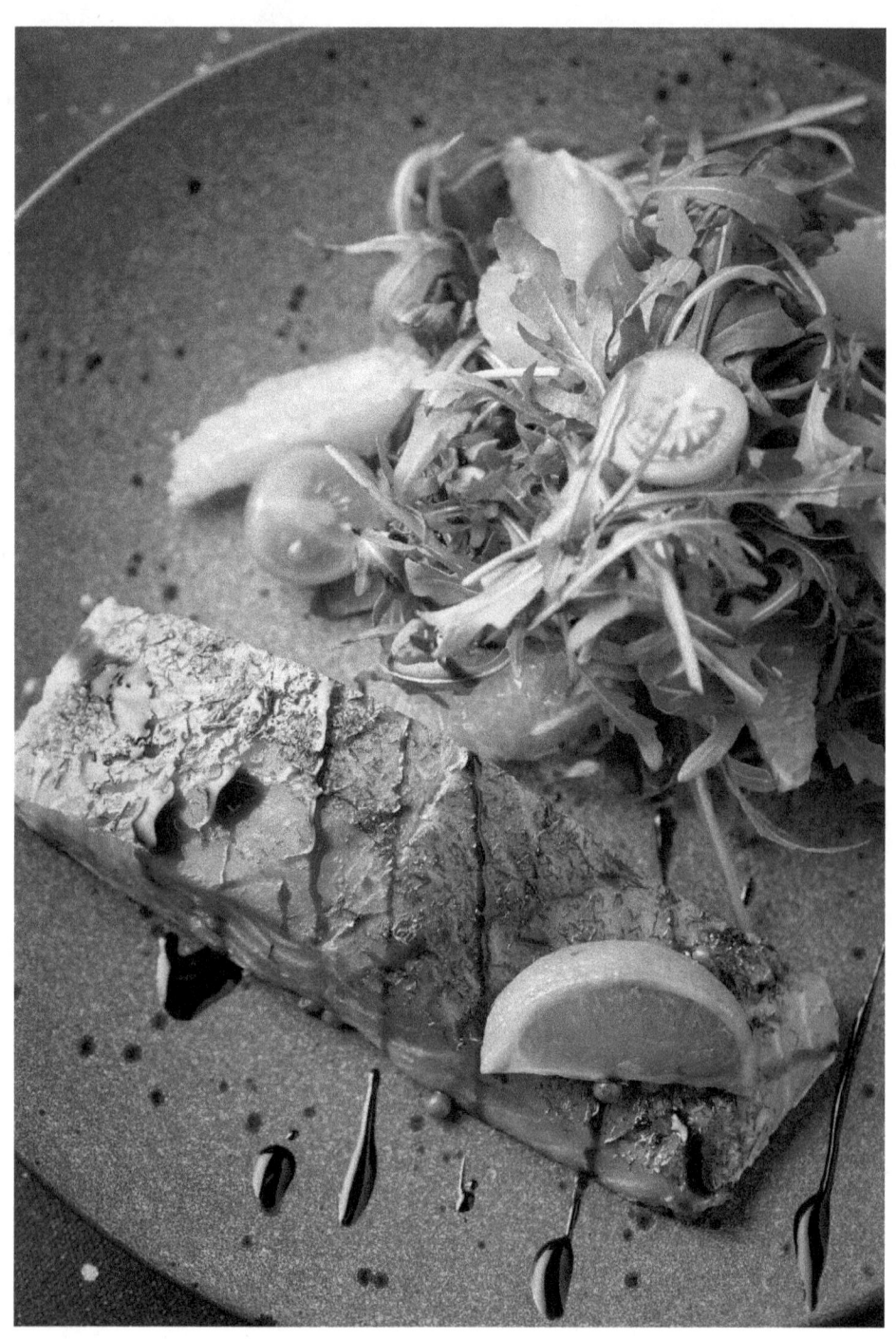

Keto Bbq Chicken Pizza Soup

Servings: 6

Cooking Time: 1 Hour 30 Minutes

Ingredients:
- 6 chicken legs
- 1 medium red onion, diced
- 4 garlic cloves
- 1 large tomato, unsweetened
- 4 cups green beans
- ¾ cup BBQ Sauce
- 1½ cups mozzarella cheese, shredded
- ¼ cup ghee
- 2 quarts water
- 2 quarts chicken stock
- Salt and black pepper, to taste
- Fresh cilantro, for garnishing

Directions:
1. Put chicken, water and salt in a large pot and bring to a boil.
2. Reduce the heat to medium-low and cook for about 75 minutes.
3. Shred the meat off the bones using a fork and keep aside.
4. Put ghee, red onions and garlic in a large soup and cook over a medium heat.

5. Add chicken stock and bring to a boil over a high heat.
6. Add green beans and tomato to the pot and cook for about 15 minutes.
7. Add BBQ Sauce, shredded chicken, salt and black pepper to the pot. 8. Ladle the soup into serving bowls and top with shredded mozzarella cheese and cilantro to serve.

Nutrition Info: Calories: 449 Carbs: 7.1g Fats: 32.5g Proteins: 30.8g Sodium: 252mg Sugar: 4.7g

Mediterranean Garden Salad

Servings: 2 Cups

Cooking Time: 5 Minutes

Ingredients:
- 6 cups mixed greens
- 2 cups cherry tomatoes, halved
- 1 medium red onion, sliced (1/2 cup)
- 3 TB. tahini paste
- 3 TB. fresh lemon juice
- 3 TB. balsamic vinegar
- 3 TB. plus 1 tsp. extra-virgin olive oil
- 3 TB. water
- 1/2 tsp. salt
- 1/2 tsp. fresh ground black pepper
- 1/2 cup pine nuts

Directions:

1. In a large bowl, add mixed greens, cherry tomatoes, and red onion.
2. In a small bowl, whisk together tahini paste, lemon juice, balsamic vinegar, 3 tablespoons extra-virgin olive oil, water, salt, and black pepper.
3. Preheat a small skillet over medium-low heat for 1 minute. Add remaining 1 teaspoon extra-virgin olive oil and pine nuts, and cook, stirring to toast evenly on all sides, for

4 minutes. Transfer pine nuts to a plate, and let cool for 2 minutes.

4. Pour dressing over vegetables, and toss to coat evenly. Top with toasted pine nuts, and serve immediately.

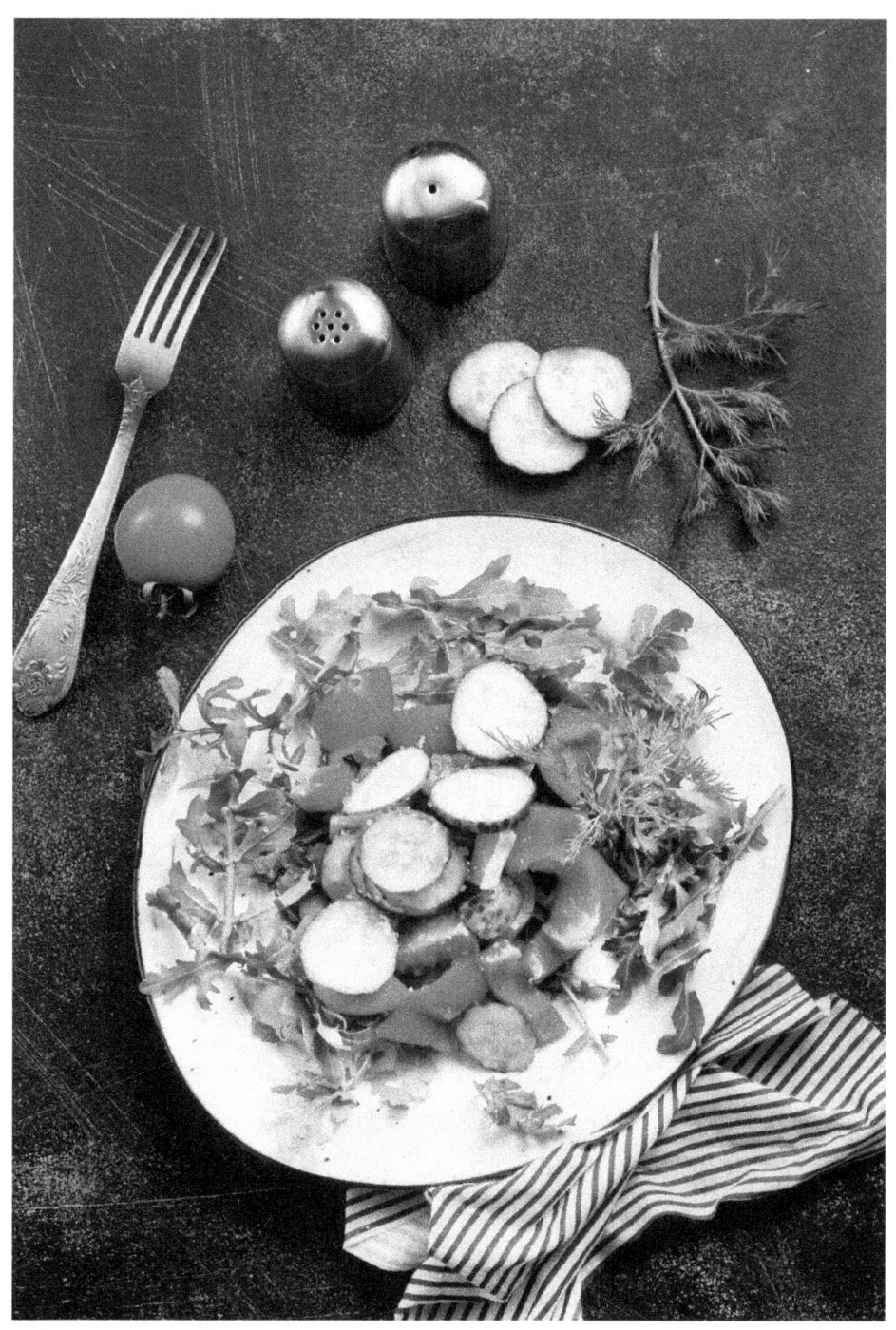

Buttery Millet

Servings: 3
Cooking Time: 15 Minutes

Ingredients:
- ¼ cup mushrooms, sliced
- ¾ cup onion, diced
- 1 tablespoon olive oil
- 1 teaspoon salt
- 3 tablespoons milk
- ½ cup millet
- 1 cup of water
- 1 teaspoon butter

Directions:
1. Pour olive oil in the skillet and add the onion.
2. Add mushrooms and roast the vegetables for 10 minutes over the medium heat. Stir them from time to time.
3. Meanwhile, pour water in the pan.
4. Add millet and salt.
5. Cook the millet with the closed lid for 15 minutes over the medium heat.
6. Then add the cooked mushroom mixture in the millet.
7. Add milk and butter. Mix up the millet well.

Nutrition Info:Per Serving:calories 198, fat 7.7, fiber 3.5, carbs 27.9, protein 4.7

Delicata Squash Soup

Servings: 5

Cooking Time: 45 minutes

Ingredients:
- 1½ cups beef bone broth
- 1small onion, peeled and grated.
- ½ teaspoon sea salt
- ¼ teaspoon poultry seasoning
- 2 small Delicata Squash, chopped
- 2 garlic cloves, minced
- 2tablespoons olive oil
- ¼ teaspoon black pepper
- 1 small lemon, juiced
- 5 tablespoons sour cream

Directions:
1. Put Delicata Squash and water in a medium pan and bring to a boil.
2. Reduce the heat and cook for about 20 minutes.
3. Drain and set aside.
4. Put olive oil, onions, garlic and poultry seasoning in a small sauce pan.
5. Cook for about 2 minutes and add broth.
6. Allow it to simmer for 5 minutes and remove from heat.

7. Whisk in the lemon juice and transfer the mixture in a blender.
8. Pulse until smooth and top with sour cream.

Nutrition Info: Calories: 109 Carbs: 4.9g Fats: 8.5g Proteins: 3g Sodium: 279mg Sugar: 2.4g

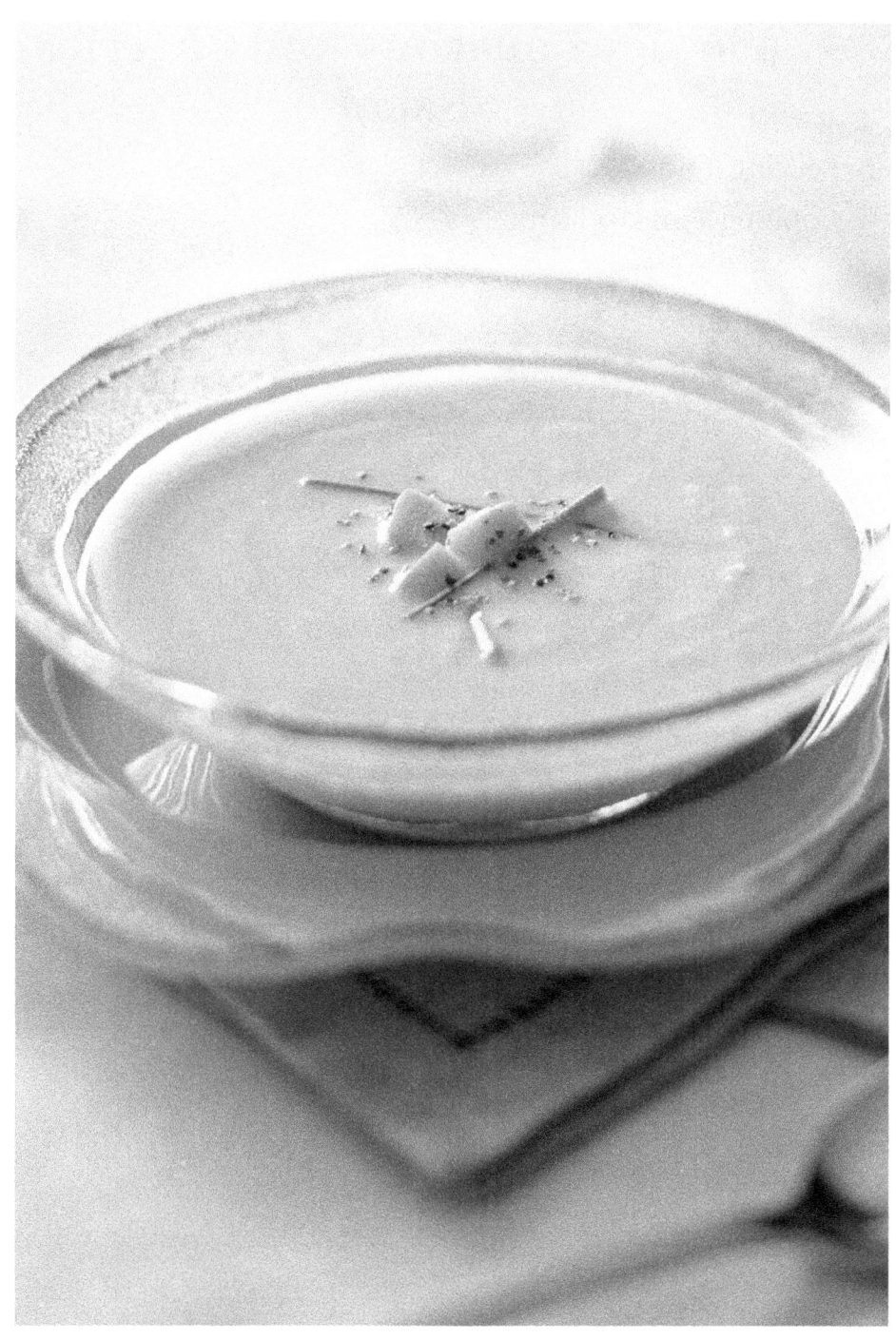

Parsley Couscous And Cherries Salad

Servings: 6

Cooking Time: 0 Minutes

Ingredients:
- 2 cups hot water
- 1 cup couscous
- ½ cup walnuts, roasted and chopped
- ½ cup cherries, pitted
- ½ cup parsley, chopped
- A pinch of sea salt and black pepper
- 1 tablespoon lime juice
- 2 tablespoons olive oil

Directions:

1. Put the couscous in a bowl, add the hot water, cover, leave aside for 10 minutes, fluff with a fork and transfer to a bowl.
2. Add the rest of the ingredients, toss and serve.

Nutrition Info: calories 200, fat 6.71, fiber 7.3, carbs 8.5, protein 5

Mint Quinoa

Servings: 8
Cooking Time: 10 Minutes

Ingredients:
- 1 cup quinoa
- 1 ¼ cup water
- 4 teaspoons lemon juice
- ¼ teaspoon garlic clove, diced
- 5 tablespoons sesame oil
- 2 cucumbers, chopped
- 1/3 teaspoon ground black pepper
- 1/3 cup tomatoes, chopped
- ½ oz scallions, chopped
- ¼ teaspoon fresh mint, chopped

Directions:
1. Pour water in the pan. Add quinoa and boil it for 10 minutes.
2. Then close the lid and let it rest for 5 minutes more.
3. Meanwhile, in the mixing bowl mix up together lemon juice, diced garlic, sesame oil, cucumbers, ground black pepper, tomatoes, scallions, and fresh mint.
4. Then add cooked quinoa and carefully mix the side dish with the help of the spoon.

5. Store tabbouleh up to 2 days in the fridge.

Nutrition Info:Per Serving:calories 168, fat 9.9, fiber 2, carbs 16.9, protein 3.6

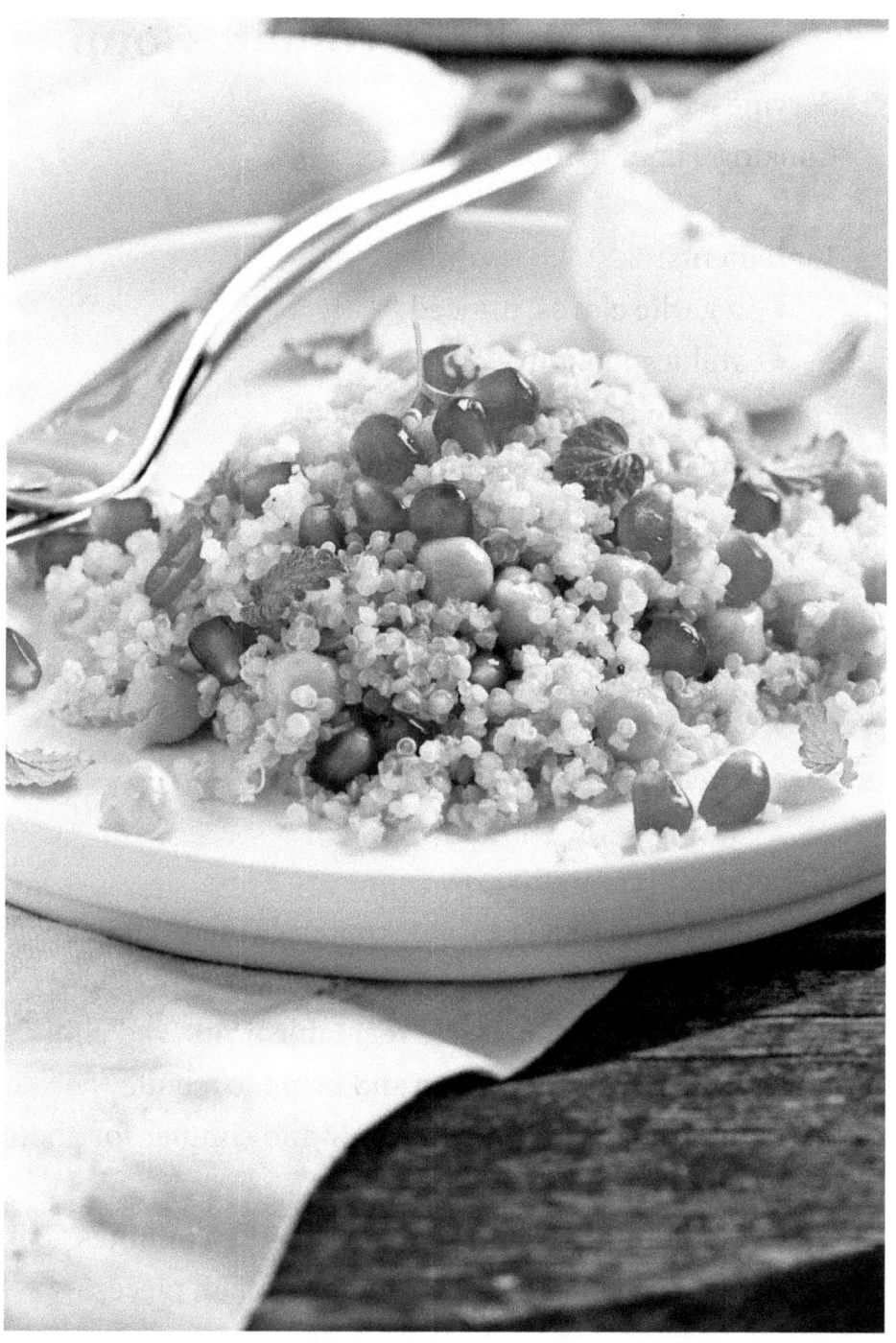

Spicy Halibut Tomato Soup

Servings: 8

Cooking Time: 1 Hour 5 minutes

Ingredients:
- 2 garlic cloves, minced
- 1tablespoonolive oil
- ¼ cup fresh parsley, chopped
- 10 anchovies canned in oil, minced
- 6 cups vegetable broth
- 1 teaspoonblack pepper
- 1 pound halibut fillets, chopped
- 3tomatoes, peeled and diced
- 1 teaspoon salt
- 1 teaspoon red chili flakes

Directions:
1. Heat olive oil in a large stockpot over medium heat and add garlic and half of the parsley.
2. Add anchovies, tomatoes, vegetable broth, red chili flakes, salt and black pepper and bring to a boil.
3. Reduce the heat to medium-low and simmer for about 20 minutes.
4. Add halibut fillets and cook for about 10 minutes.
5. Dish out the halibut and shred into small pieces.

6. Mix back with the soup and garnish with the remaining fresh parsley to serve.

Nutrition Info: Calories: 170 Carbs: 3g Fats: 6.7g Proteins: 23.4g Sodium: 2103mg Sugar: 1.8g

Beans With Pancetta, Sage, And Vinegar

Servings: 6
Cooking Time: 15 Minutes

Ingredients:
- 1 red onion, finely chopped
- 1/4 cup fresh continental parsley, chopped
- 2 cans (400 g each) borlotti beans, rinsed, and drained
- 2 garlic cloves, finely chopped
- 3 anchovy fillets, drained, finely chopped
- 3 fresh sage leaves, chopped
- 50 g pancetta, finely chopped
- 60 ml (about 1/4 cup) red wine vinegar
- 60 ml (about 1/4 cup) water
- 80 ml (about 1/3 cup) extra-virgin olive oil
- Fresh continental parsley leaves, plus more to serve
- Red wine vinegar, plus more, to serve

Directions:
1. In a heavy-bottomed saucepan, heat the oil over medium-low heat. Add the garlic, onion, pancetta, and the anchovy; cook for about 8 minutes, stirring often, until the onion is soft.

2. Add the water, vinegar, and the sage. Adjust the heat to medium-high; bring to a simmer, cooking for about 3 minutes or until the liquid is slightly reduced. Transfer into a bowl. Stir in the beans and set aside; letting the mixture cool completely.

3. Season the mixture with more salt, pepper, and vinegar. Stir in the parsley, transfer into a serving bowl, top with the parsley, and serve.

4. Make-ahead: Prepare the ingredients up to step 2 up to 1 day ahead before serving day; cover and store in the refrigerator. Four hours before serving, remove from the fridge. Continue from step 3 thirty minutes before serving.

Nutrition Info:Per Serving:245 cal, 14 g total fat (1 g sat. fat), 19 g carb, 9 g protein, 579.84 mg sodium, 1 g sugar, 6 mg chol., and 6 g fiber.

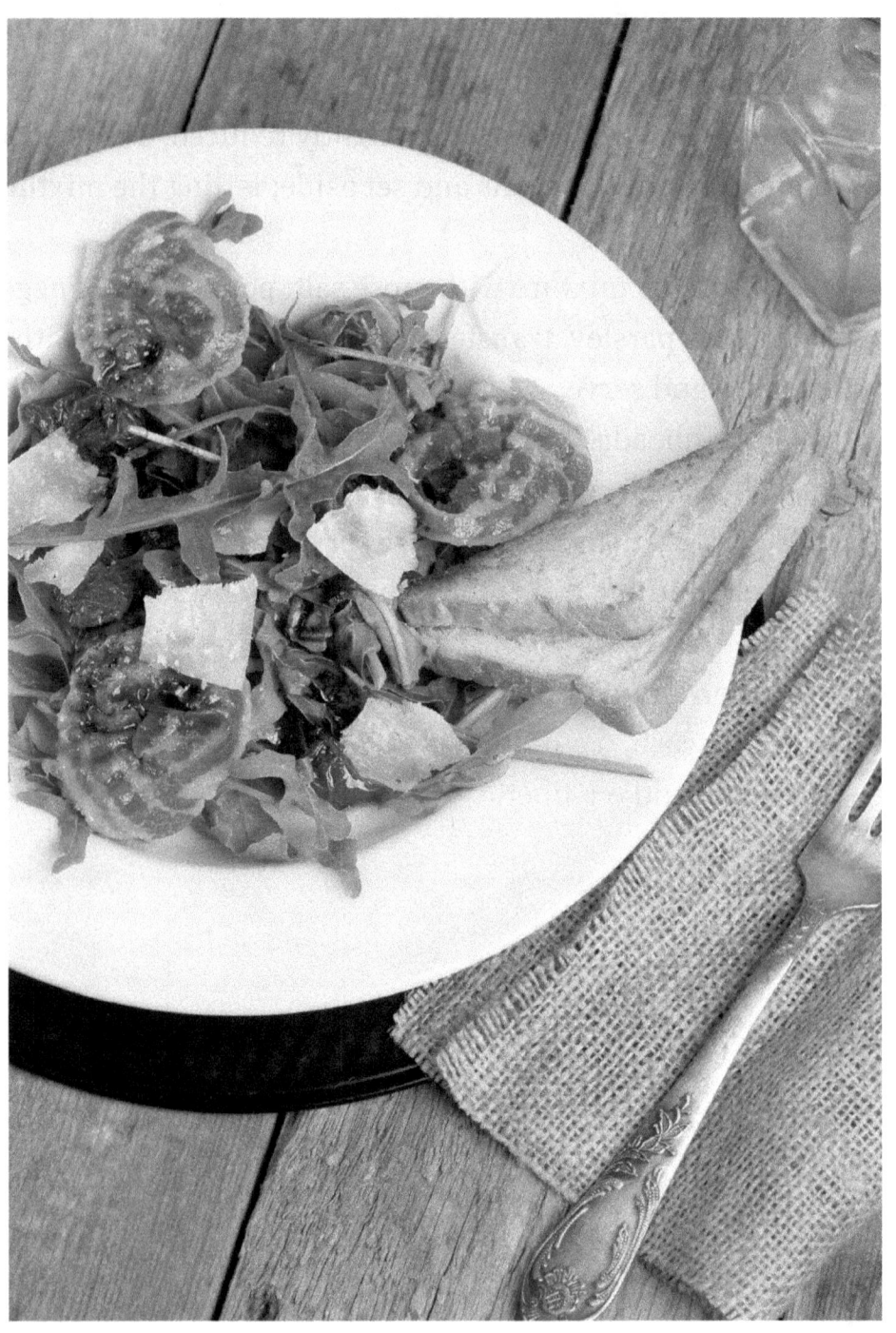

Mediterranean-style Vegetable Stew

Servings: 4

Cooking Time: 15 Minutes

Ingredients:
- 1 can (14 ounces) cannellini beans, rinsed, drained
- 1 red onion, peeled, chopped
- 1 tablespoon cilantro, chopped
- 2 cloves garlic, peeled, crushed
- 2 small zucchini, thinly sliced
- 2 tablespoons lemon juice
- 2 tablespoons olive oil, divided
- 3 tomatoes, quartered
- 4 cups vegetable stock
- 5 ounces carrots, peeled, cut into ribbons using a vegetable peeler 8 ounces turnips, peeled, chopped
- Crusty whole-wheat bread, to serve
- Lemon wedges, to serve

Directions:

1. In a large-sized pot, heat 1 tablespoons of the olive oil. Add the garlic, onion, and turnip; sauté for 5 minutes. Add the carrots, tomatoes, zucchini;
sauté for 2 minutes.

2. Add the stock, the lemon juice, the beans, and the remaining oil; season to taste. Bring to a boil; simmer for 3

to 4 minutes. Sprinkle with cilantro. Serve with the bread and the lemon wedges.

Nutrition Info:Per Serving:190 cal., 11 g total fat (1 g sat. fat), 0 mg chol., 1020 mg sodium, 1000 mg potassium, 29 g carb, 9 g fiber, 16 g sugar, 5 g protein, 160% vitamin A, 140% vitamin C, 10% calcium, and 8% iron.

Cheesy Potatoes

Servings: 4
Cooking Time: 20 Minutes

Ingredients:
- 4 sweet potatoes
- ¼ cup Cheddar cheese, shredded
- 2 teaspoons butter
- 1 tablespoon fresh parsley, chopped
- ½ teaspoon salt

Directions:
1. Make the lengthwise cut in every sweet potato and bake them for 10 minutes at 360F.
2. After this, scoop ½ part of every sweet potato flesh.
3. Fill the vegetables with salt, parsley, butter, and shredded cheese.
4. Return the sweet potatoes in the oven back and bake them for 10 minutes more at 355F.

Nutrition Info:Per Serving:calories 47, fat 4.3, fiber 0.1, carbs 0.4, protein 1.8

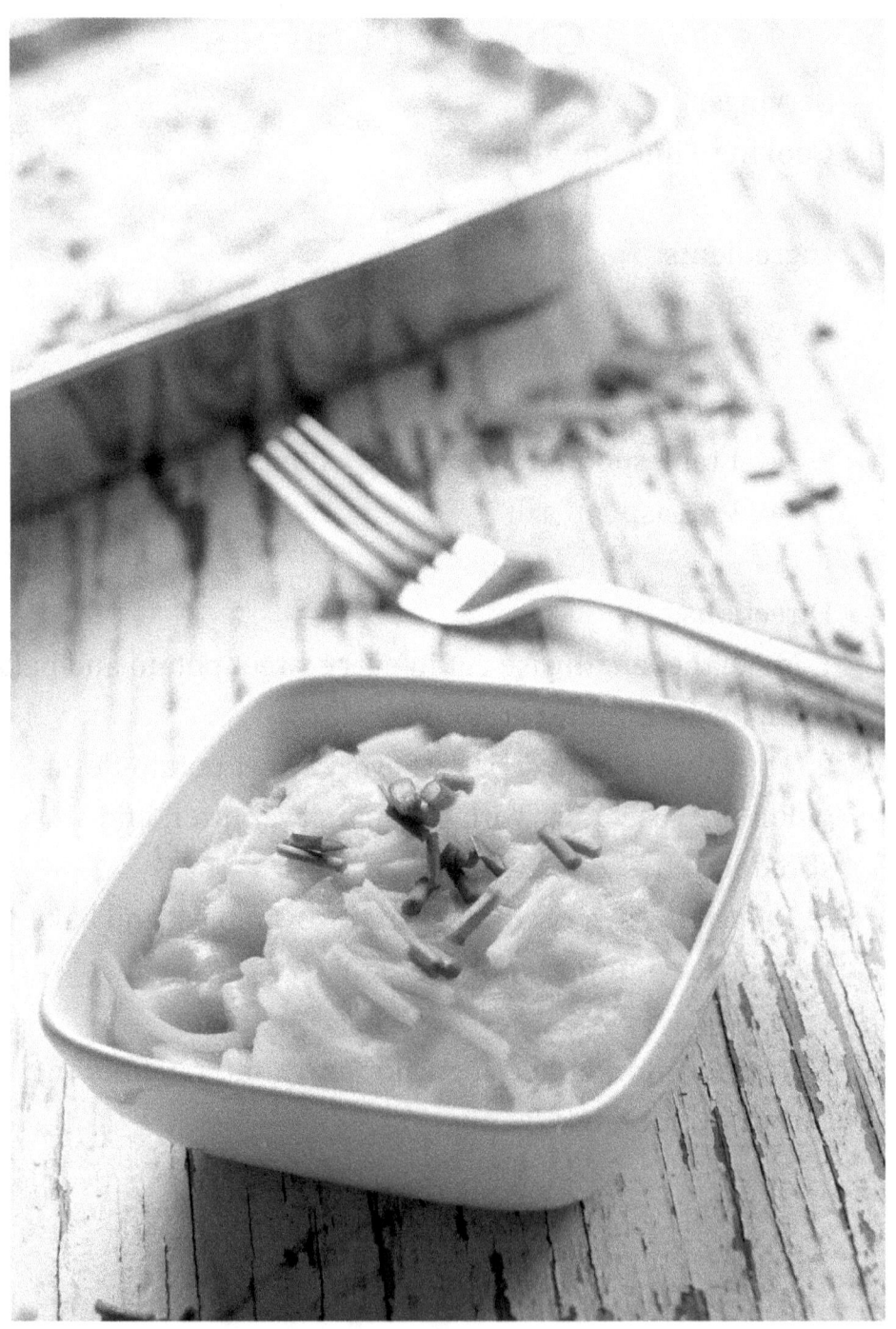

Greek Beets

Servings: 2

Cooking Time: 25 Minutes

Ingredients:
- 1 beet, trimmed
- 1/3 teaspoon minced garlic
- 2 tablespoons walnuts
- 2 tablespoons Greek yogurt

Directions:
1. Preheat the oven to 360F.
2. Place the beet in the tray and bake it for 25 minutes. The baked beet should be tender.
3. Let the beet chill a little. Peel it.
4. After this, grate it with the help of the grated and transfer in the bowl.
5. Add walnuts, Greek yogurt, and minced garlic. Mix up the mixture well.
6. Place it in the fridge for at least 10 minutes before serving.

Nutrition Info:Per Serving:calories 79, fat 4.8, fiber 1.5, carbs 6.4, protein 3.9

Snow Peas Salad

Servings: 4

Cooking Time: 10 Minutes

Ingredients:
- 3 cups snow peas, trimmed
- 1 and ¼ cup bean sprouts
- 1 tablespoon basil, chopped
- 1 tablespoon lime juice
- 1 teaspoon ginger, grated
- 2 spring onions, chopped
- 2 garlic cloves, minced

Directions:

1. Put the snow peas in a pot, add water to cover, bring to a simmer and cook over medium heat for 10 minutes.
2. Drain the peas, transfer them to a bowl, add the sprouts and the rest of the ingredients, toss and keep in the fridge for 6 hours before serving.

Nutrition Info: calories 200, fat 8.6, fiber 3, carbs 5.4, protein 3.4

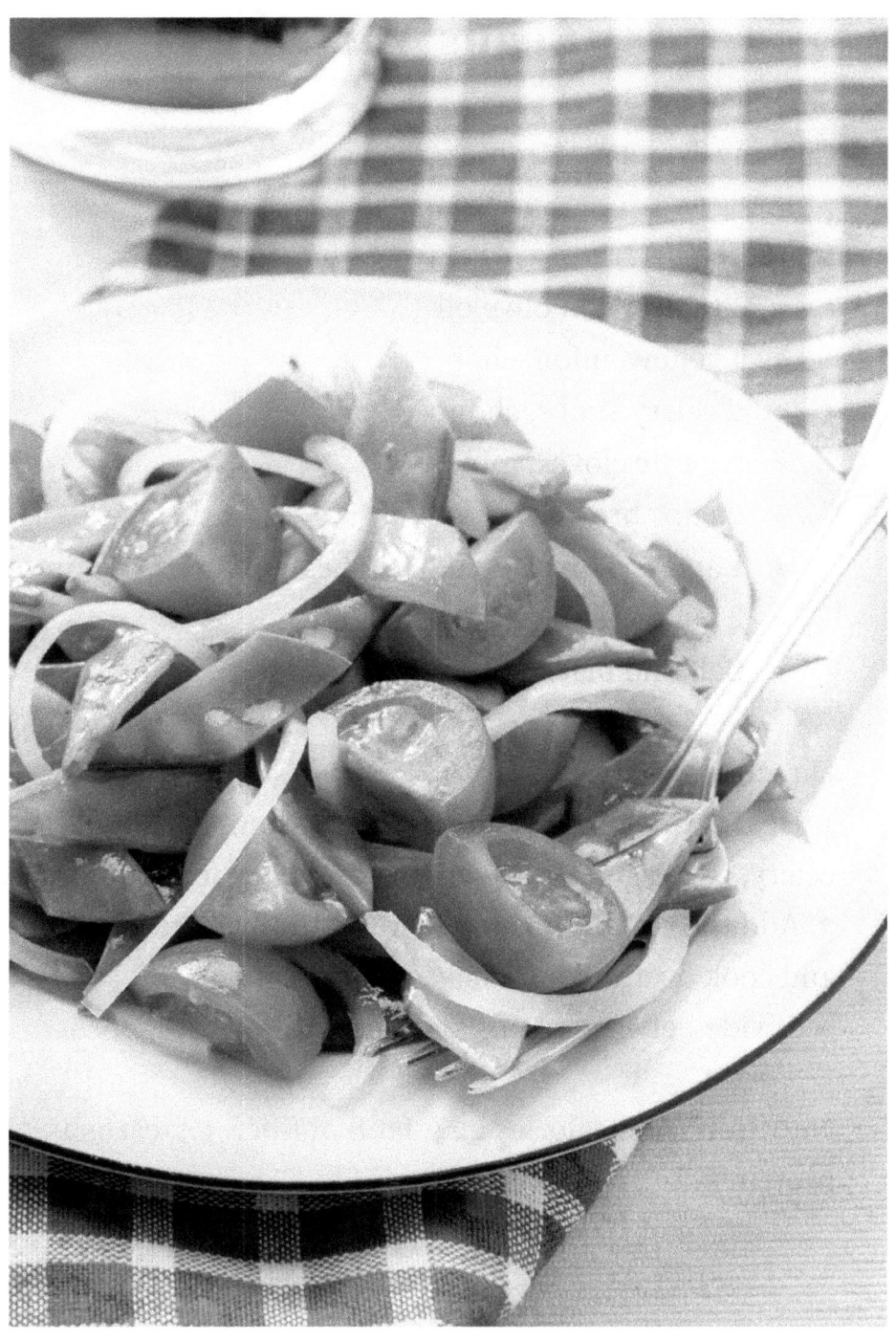

Beans And Rice

Servings: 6

Cooking Time: 55 Minutes

Ingredients:
- 1 tablespoon olive oil
- 1 yellow onion, chopped
- 2 celery stalks, chopped
- 2 garlic cloves, minced
- 2 cups brown rice
- 1 and ½ cup canned black beans, rinsed and drained
- 4 cups water
- Salt and black pepper to the taste

Directions:
1. Heat up a pan with the oil over medium heat, add the celery, garlic and the onion, stir and cook for 10 minutes.
2. Add the rest of the ingredients, stir, bring to a simmer and cook over medium heat for 45 minutes.
3. Divide between plates and serve.

Nutrition Info: calories 224, fat 8.4, fiber 3.4, carbs 15.3, protein 6.2

Parsley Tomato Mix

Servings: 4

Cooking Time: 10 Minutes

Ingredients:
- 4 medium tomatoes, roughly cubed
- 1 garlic clove, minced
- 1 tablespoon olive oil
- ½ teaspoon sweet paprika
- Salt and black pepper to the taste
- ½ bunch parsley, chopped

Directions:
1. Heat up a pot with the olive oil over medium heat, add the tomatoes and the garlic and sauté for 5 minutes.
2. Add the rest of the ingredients, toss, cook for 3-4 minutes more, divide into bowls and serve.

Nutrition Info: calories 220, fat 9.4, fiber 5.3, carbs 6.5, protein 4.6

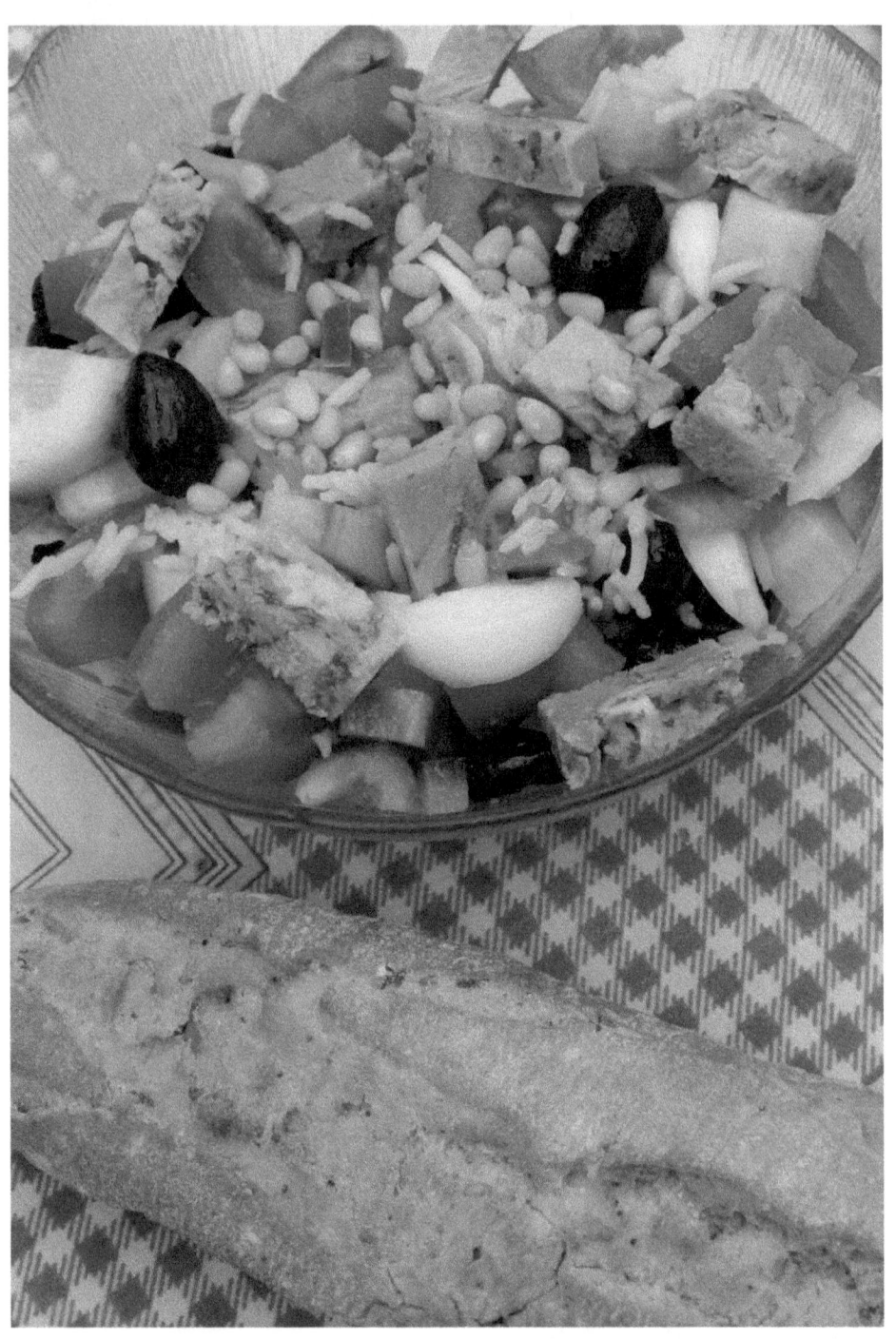

Lemon Chili Cucumbers

Servings: 3

Cooking Time: 30 Minutes

Ingredients:
- 3 cucumbers
- 3 tablespoons lemon juice
- ¾ teaspoon lemon zest
- 3 teaspoons dill, chopped
- 1 tablespoon olive oil
- ¾ teaspoon chili flakes

Directions:
1. Peel the cucumbers and chop them roughly.
2. Place the cucumbers in the big glass jar.
3. Add lemon zest, lemon juice, dill, olive oil, and chili flakes.
4. Close the lid and shake well.
5. Marinate the cucumbers for 30 minutes.

Nutrition Info:Per Serving:calories 92, fat 5.2, fiber 1.8, carbs 11.9, protein 2.3

Tuna-dijon Salad

Servings: 6

Cooking Time: Minutes

Ingredients:
- 5 whole small radishes, stems removed and chopped
- 3 stalks green onions, chopped
- 1 cup chopped parsley leaves
- ½ cup chopped fresh mint leaves, stems removed
- Six slices heirloom tomatoes for serving
- Pita chips or pita pockets for serving
- 2 1/2 celery stalks, chopped
- 1/2 English cucumber, chopped
- 1/2 medium-sized red onion, finely chopped
- 1/2 cup pitted Kalamata olives, halved
- 3 5-ounce cans Genova tuna in olive oil
- 1 1/2 limes, juice of
- 1/2 tsp crushed red pepper flakes, optional
- 1/2 tsp sumac
- 1/3 cup Early Harvest extra virgin olive oil
- 2 1/2 tsp good quality Dijon mustard
- Pinch of salt and pepper
- Zest of 1 lime

Directions:

1. Make the dressing by mixing all ingredients in a small bowl until thoroughly blended. Set aside to allow flavors to mix.
2. In a large salad bowl, make the salad.
3. Mix well mint leaves, parsley. Olives, chopped veggies, and tuna.
4. Drizzle with vinaigrette and toss well to coat.
5. Put in the fridge for at least half an hour to allow flavors to mix.
6. Toss again. Top with tomatoes.
7. Serve with pita chips on the side and enjoy.

Nutrition Info: Calories per Serving: 299; Carbs: 6.6g; Protein: 25.7g; Fats: 19.2g

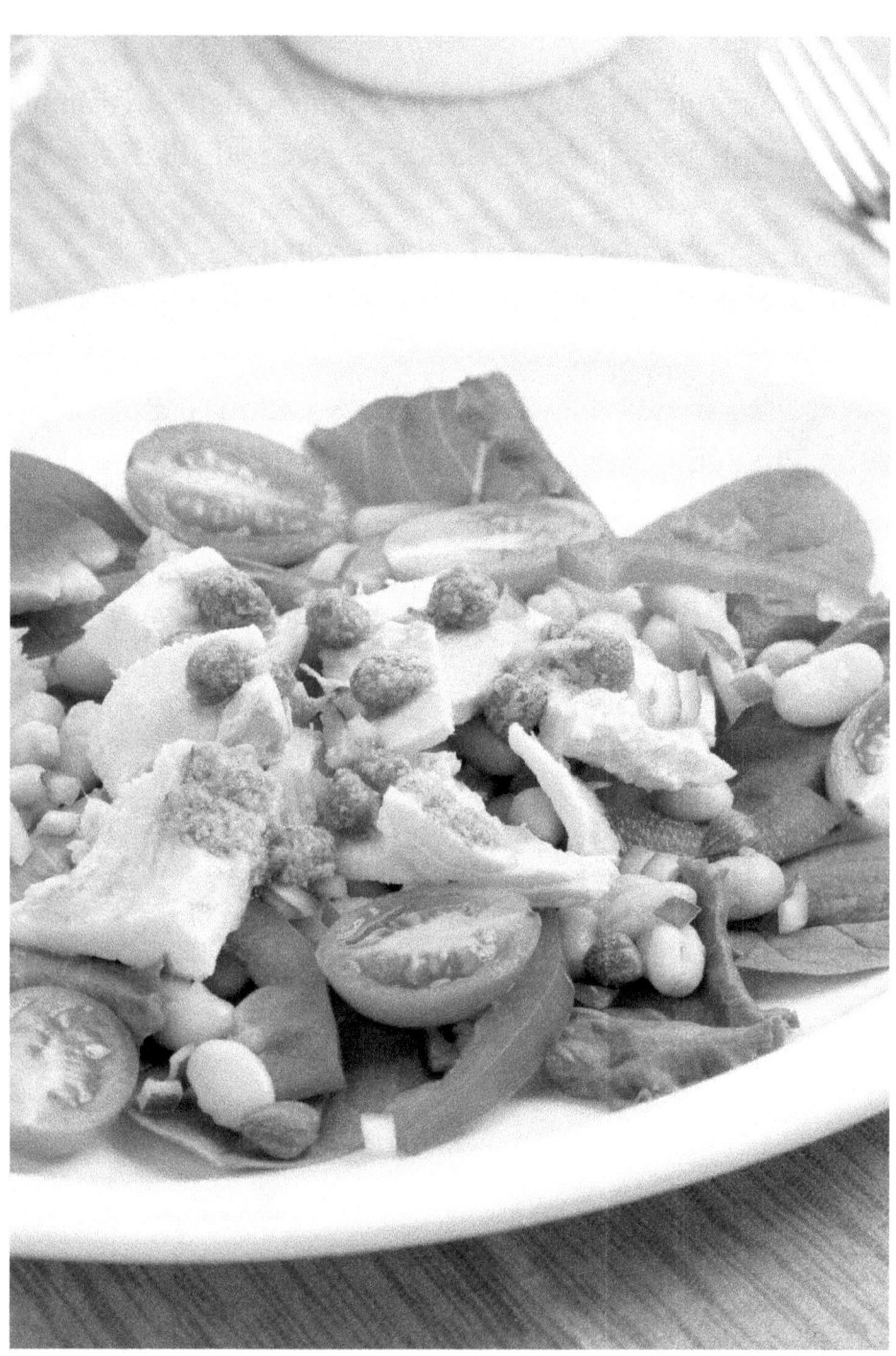

Grilled Chicken Salad

Servings: 4

Cooking Time: 30 Minutes

Ingredients:
- 2 chicken fillets
- 1 teaspoon dried oregano
- 1 teaspoon dried basil
- 2 tablespoons olive oil
- 2 cups arugula leaves
- 1 cup cherry tomatoes, halved
- ¼ cup green olives
- 1 cucumber, sliced
- 1 lemon, juiced
- 2 tablespoons extra virgin olive oil
- Salt and pepper to taste

Directions:

1. Season the chicken with salt, pepper, oregano and basil then drizzle it with olive oil.
2. Heat a grill pan over medium flame then place the chicken on the grill. Cook on each side until browned then cut into thin strips.
3. Combine the chicken with the rest of the ingredients and mix gently.

4. Adjust the taste with salt and pepper and serve the salad as fresh as possible.

Nutrition Info: Per Serving:Calories: 280 Fat: 19.5g Protein: 21.6g Carbohydrates: 6.4g

Chili Cabbage And Coconut

Servings: 4

Cooking Time: 20 Minutes

Ingredients:
- 3 tablespoons olive oil
- 1 sprig curry leaves, chopped
- 1 teaspoon mustard seeds, crushed
- 1 green cabbage head, shredded
- 4 green chili peppers, chopped
- ½ cup coconut flesh, grated
- Salt and black pepper to the taste

Directions:
1. Heat up a pan with the oil over medium heat, add the curry leaves, mustard seeds and the chili peppers and cook for 5 minutes.
2. Add the rest of the ingredients, toss and cook for 15 minutes more.
3. Divide the mix between plates and serve as a side dish.

Nutrition Info: calories 221, fat 5.5, fiber 11.1, carbs 22.1, protein 6.7

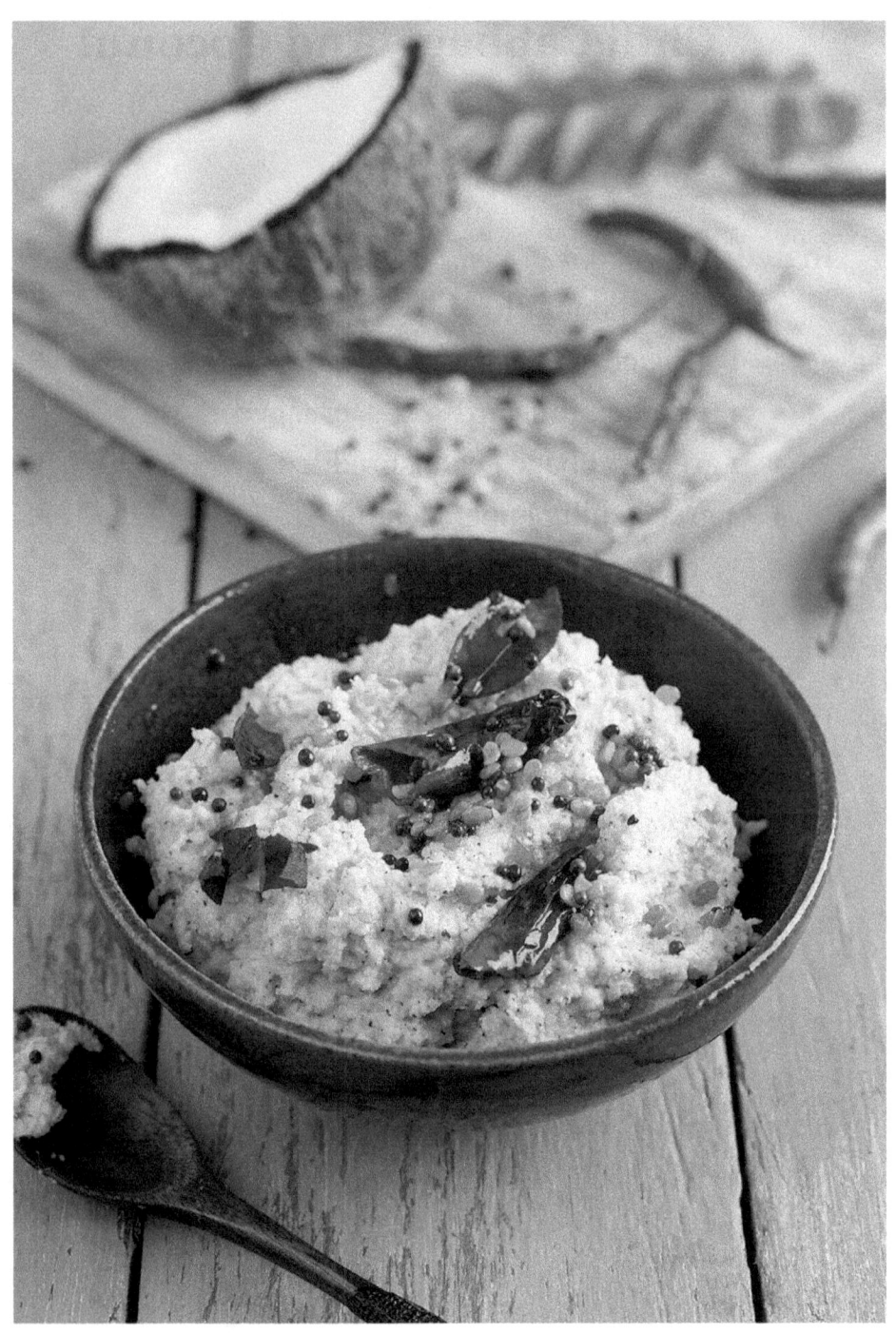

Spinach And Cranberry Salad

Servings: 4

Cooking Time: 5 Minutes

Ingredients:
- ¼ cup cider vinegar
- ¼ cup honey
- ¼ cup white wine vinegar
- ¼ tsp paprika
- ½ cup olive oil
- ½ cup pumpkin seeds
- 1 cup dried cranberries
- 1 lb spinach, rinsed and torn into bite sized pieces
- 2 tsp minced onion

Directions:

1. Toast pumpkin seeds by placing in a nonstick saucepan on medium fire. Stir frequently and toast for at least 3 to 5 minutes. Remove from fire and set aside.
2. In a medium bowl, mix well olive oil, cider vinegar, white wine vinegar, paprika, onion, and honey. Whisk well until mixture is uniform.
3. In a large salad bowl, add torn spinach.
4. Drizzle with dressing and toss well to coat.
5. Garnish with cooled and toasted pumpkin seeds and dried cranberries.

6. Serve and enjoy.

Nutrition Info: Calories per Serving: 531.3; Fat: 34.9g; Protein: 9.1g; Carbs: 45.2g

Dill Cucumber Salad

Servings: 8
Cooking Time: 0 Minutes

Ingredients:
- 4 cucumbers, sliced
- 1 cup white wine vinegar
- 2 white onions, sliced
- 1 tablespoon dill, chopped

Directions:
1. In a bowl, mix the cucumber with the onions, vinegar and the dill, toss well and keep in the fridge for 1 hour before serving as a side salad.

Nutrition Info: calories 182, fat 3.5, fiber 4.5, carbs 8.5, protein 4.5

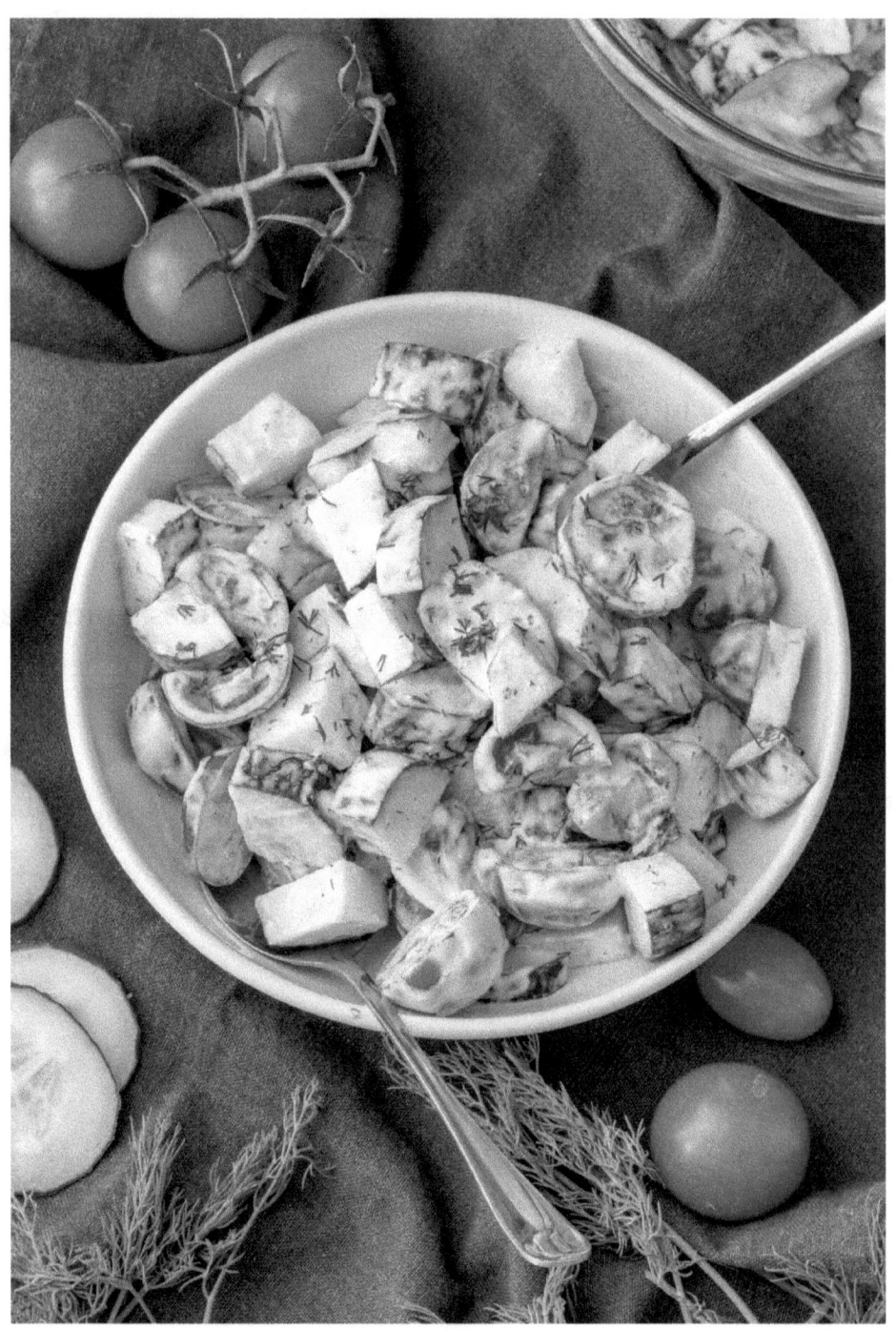

Nutty, Curry-citrus Garden Salad

Servings: 2

Cooking Time: 0 Minutes

Ingredients:
- ¼ tsp curry powder
- 1 medium carrot, shredded
- 1 tsp Balsamic vinegar
- 2 cups spring mix salad greens
- 2 tbsp orange juice
- 2 tsp extra virgin olive oil
- 8 pecan halves, chopped
- Pepper and salt to taste

Directions:
1. In a small bowl, whisk well curry powder, balsamic vinegar, olive oil, and orange juice.
2. Season with pepper and salt to taste. Mix well.
3. In a salad bowl, mix shredded carrot and salad greens.
4. Pour in dressing, toss well to coat.
5. To serve, top with chopped pecans and enjoy.

Nutrition Info: Calories per serving: 117; Protein: 2.39g; Carbs: 10.2g; Fat: 7.4g

Mouthwatering Steakhouse Salad

Servings: 4
Cooking Time: 30 Minutes

Ingredients:
- ½ tsp pepper
- ½ tsp salt
- 1 lb. green beans, trimmed
- 10oz timed filet mignon
- 2 garlic cloves
- 2 tsp extra virgin olive oil
- 3 tbsp balsamic vinegar
- 4 medium red bell peppers, seeded and halved
- 6 medium tomatoes cut into ¼ wedges
- 8 cups mesclun

Directions:
1. Preheat the grill or the broiler. Put the red peppers on the grill and cook until the skin blisters and chars. Peel away blackened skins and cut into chunks.
2. Meanwhile, lay the filet mignon on a cutting board and slit it lengthwise until it opens like a book when pressed flat. Sprinkle with ¼ teaspoon salt and ¼ teaspoon pepper. Cut 1 garlic clove and rub the cut sides all over the steak. Grill the beef until done. Slice it thinly and set aside.

3. In a saucepan, cook the beans in the boiling water until tender. Drain and rinse with cold water. Set aside.
4. Mince the remaining garlic and add to vinegar, oil and shallot. Season with salt and pepper.
5. In a plate, prepare a mesclun bead and arrange the steak, beans, tomatoes and red peppers on top. Drizzle with the dressing. Serve warm.

Nutrition Info:Calories per serving 220.3; Protein: 21.6g; Carbs: 21.1g; Fat: 5.5g

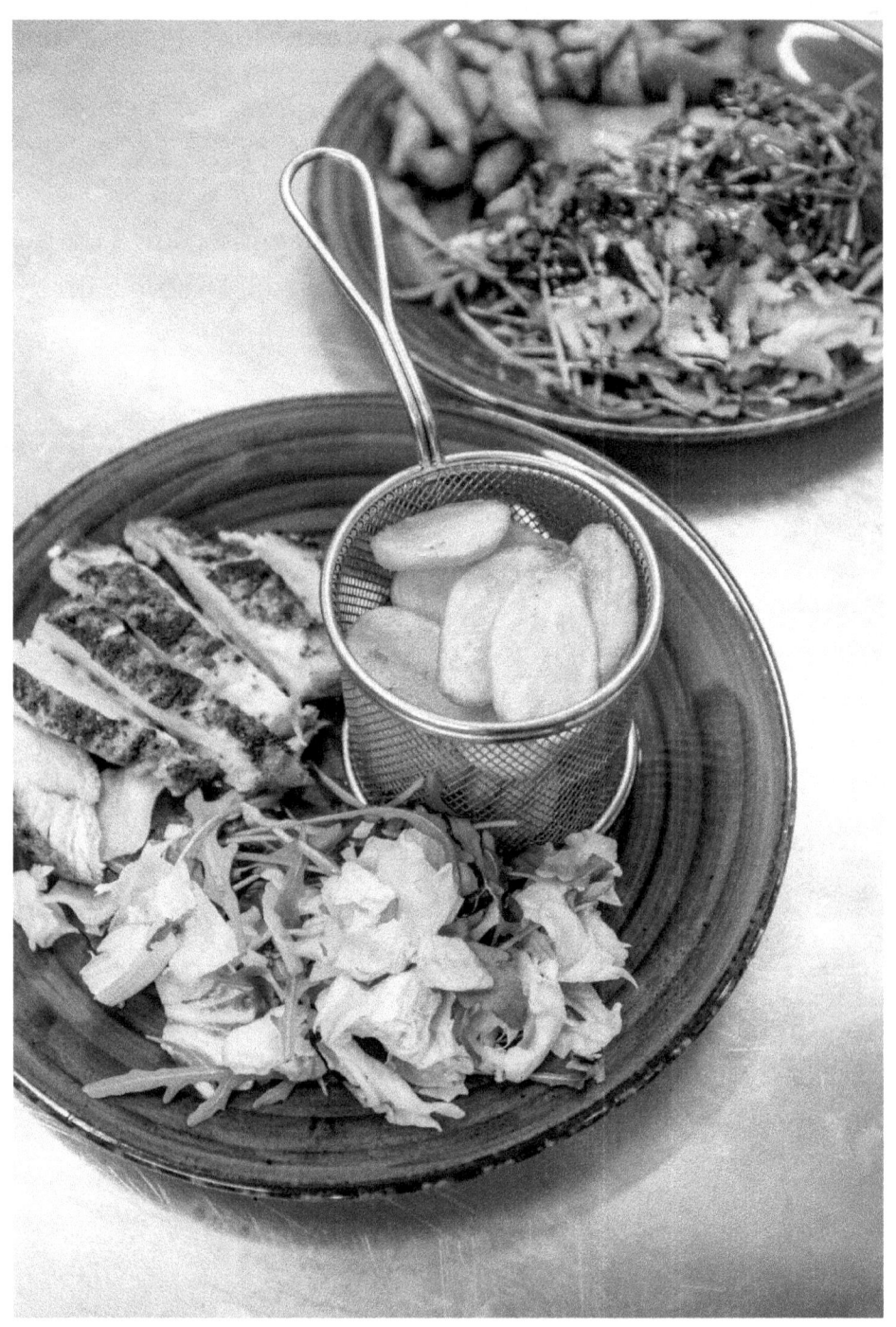

Green Beans With Pomegranate Dressing

Servings: 8
Cooking Time: 30 Minutes

Ingredients:
- 1 small red onion, sliced into half moons
- 1 teaspoon cinnamon
- 2 red pepper, cut into quarters
- 200 g feta cheese, drained, crumbled
- 200 g green beans, blanched (frozen beans preferred)
- 3 medium aubergine or eggplant, cut into chunks, or 15 small, halved 6 tablespoons extra-virgin olive oil
- Handful parsley, roughly chopped
- Seeds of 1 pomegranate
- 5 tablespoons extra-virgin olive oil
- 2 tablespoons pomegranate molasses
- 1 tablespoon lemon juice
- 1 small garlic clove, crushed

Directions:
1. Heat the oven to 200C, gas to 6, or fan to 180C. Preheat the grill to the highest setting.
2. With the skin side up, place them in a baking sheet; grill until blackened. Place in a plastic bag, seal, and let rest for

5 minutes. When cool enough to handle, scrape the blackened skins off, discard, the set aside the peppers.

3. Place the aubergine chunks into a baking tray; drizzle with the olive oil, sprinkle with the cinnamon, and season with the salt and pepper. Roast for about 25 minutes, or until softened and golden.

4. Meanwhile, in a bowl, combine all the dressing ingredients until well mixed.

5. To serve:

6. Place the green beans, aubergine chunks, peppers, and onion into a large-sized serving platter. Scatter the feta and the pomegranate seeds over the vegetables. Drizzle the dressing and top with parsley.

Nutrition Info:Per Serving:258 cal, 21 g fat (5 g sat. fat), 12 g carbs, 11 g sugars, 0 g fiber, 6 g protein, and 0.94 g sodium.

Cauliflower And Thyme Soup

Servings: 6

Cooking Time: 30 Minutes

Ingredients:
- 2 teaspoons thyme powder
- 1 head cauliflower
- 3 cups vegetable stock
- ½ teaspoon matcha green tea powder
- 3 tablespoons olive oil
- Salt and black pepper, to taste
- 5 garlic cloves, chopped

Directions:
1. Put the vegetable stock, thyme and matcha powder to a large pot over medium-high heat and bring to a boil.
2. Add cauliflower and cook for about 10 minutes.
3. Meanwhile, put the olive oil and garlic in a small sauce pan and cook for about 1 minute.
4. Add the garlic, salt and black pepper and cook for about 2 minutes.
5. Transfer into an immersion blender and blend until smooth.
6. Dish out and serve immediately.

Nutrition Info: Calories: 79 Carbs: 3.8g Fats: 7.1g Proteins: 1.3g Sodium: 39mg Sugar: 1.5g

Turkey Maghiritsa

Servings: 6
Cooking Time: 20 Minutes

Ingredients:
- 1 1/2 cups leftover cooked turkey, shredded (lean meat preferred, but you can use light and dark meat)
- 1 cup cooked whole-grain rice
- 1 cup romaine lettuce, shredded
- 1 tablespoon fresh dill, chopped
- 1/2 cup sliced green onions
- 1/2 teaspoon whole-wheat flour
- 1/2 teaspoon freshly squeezed lemon juice
- 1/4 teaspoon freshly ground black pepper
- 1/4 teaspoon salt
- 2 1/2 cups onion, finely chopped
- 2 large eggs
- 2 tablespoons freshly squeezed lemon juice
- 2 tablespoons olive oil
- 7 cups chicken broth, fat-free, less-sodium divided
- Dash of salt

Directions:
1. In a bowl, whisk the flour and 2 tablespoons lemon juice until smooth. Add the eggs; whisk until smooth.

2. In a medium-sized saucepan, bring 1 cup of the broth into a simmer over medium-high heat. Gradually add the hot broth into the egg mixture, constantly stirring with a whisk. Return the egg mixture into the saucepan; cook for 2 minutes, constantly whisking, until slightly thick. Remove from the heat and set aside.

3. In a large-sized saucepan, heat the olive oil over medium-high heat. Add the onion and the dash of salt; sauté for about 8 minutes or until tender. Add the remaining 6 cups of broth; bring to a boil. When boiling, reduce the heat to a simmer; cook for 5 minutes more. Add the turkey; simmer for 2

minutes. Add the rice and slowly whisk in the egg mixture. Keep the soup warm over low heat. When ready to serve, add the remaining ingredients.

Nutrition Info:Per Serving:232 Cal, 9.1 g total fat (1.9 g sat. fat, 4.9 g mono fat, 1.3 g poly fat), 18 g protein, 17g carb, 2 g fiber, 98 g chol., 1.5 mg iron, 697 mg sodium, and 34 mg calcium.

Quinoa And Greens Salad

Servings: 4
Cooking Time: 0 Minutes

Ingredients:
- 1 cup quinoa, cooked
- 1 medium bunch collard greens, chopped
- 4 tablespoons walnuts, chopped
- 2 tablespoons balsamic vinegar
- 4 tablespoons tahini paste
- 4 tablespoons cold water
- A pinch of salt and black pepper
- 1 tablespoon olive oil

Directions:
1. In a bowl, mix the tahini with the water and vinegar and whisk.
2. In a bowl, mix the quinoa with the rest of the ingredients and the tahini dressing, toss, divide the mix between plates and serve as a side dish.

Nutrition Info: calories 175, fat 3, fiber 3, carbs 5, protein 3

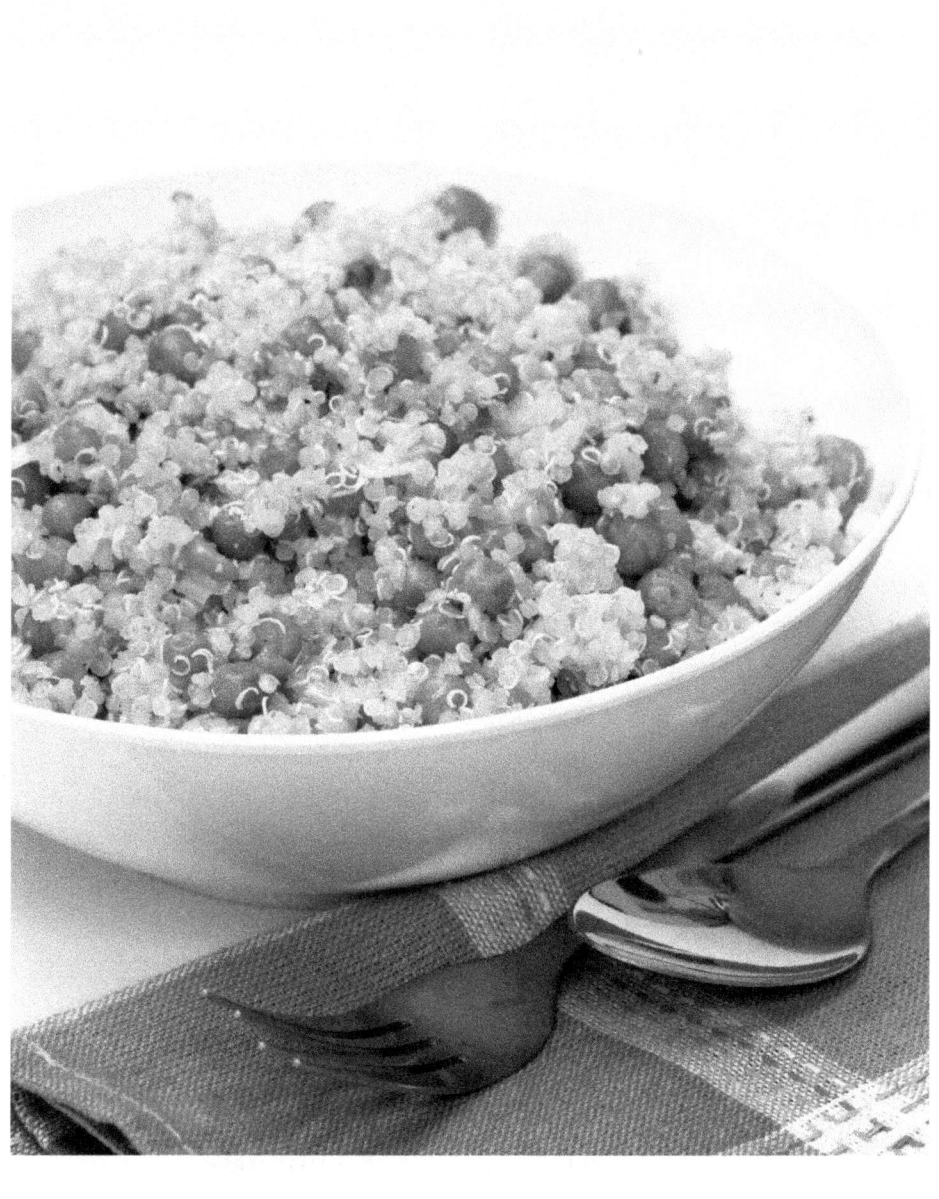

Mushroom Spinach Soup

Servings: 4

Cooking Time: 25 Minutes

Ingredients:
- 1 cup spinach, cleaned and chopped
- 100 g mushrooms, chopped
- 1 onion
- 6 garlic cloves
- ½ teaspoon red chili powder
- Salt and black pepper, to taste
- 3 tablespoons buttermilk
- 1 teaspoon almond flour
- 2 cups chicken broth
- 3 tablespoons butter
- ¼ cup fresh cream, for garnish

Directions:
1. Heat butter in a pan and add onions and garlic.
2. Sauté for about 3 minutes and add spinach, salt and red chili powder.
3. Sauté for about 4 minutes and add mushrooms.
4. Transfer into a blender and blend to make a puree.
5. Return to the pan and add buttermilk and almond flour for creamy texture.
6. Mix well and simmer for about 2 minutes.

7. Garnish with fresh cream and serve hot.

Nutrition Info: Calories: 160 Carbs: 7g Fats: 13.3g Proteins: 4.7g Sodium: 462mg Sugar: 2.7g

Spicy Herb Potatoes (batata Harra)

Servings: 1 Cup
Cooking Time: 25 Minutes

Ingredients:
- 15 small new red potatoes (11/2 lb.), scrubbed and dried
- 1 tsp. salt
- 4 TB. extra-virgin olive oil
- 3 TB. minced garlic
- 1 cup fresh cilantro, finely chopped
- 1/2 tsp. cayenne
- 1/2 tsp. black pepper

Directions:
1. Preheat the oven to 425°F.
2. Cut red potatoes into 1-inch pieces. Add potatoes to a large bowl, and toss with salt and 3 tablespoons extra-virgin olive oil.
3. Spread potatoes in an even layer on a baking sheet, and bake for 20 to 25 minutes or until golden. Remove from the oven, and let stand for 5 minutes.
4. Using a spatula, transfer potatoes to a large serving bowl.

5. Heat a small saucepan over low heat. Add remaining 1 tablespoon extra virgin olive oil and garlic, and sauté for 3 minutes. Add garlic to potatoes.

6. Add cilantro, cayenne, and black pepper to potatoes, and gently toss to combine.

7. Serve warm or at room temperature.

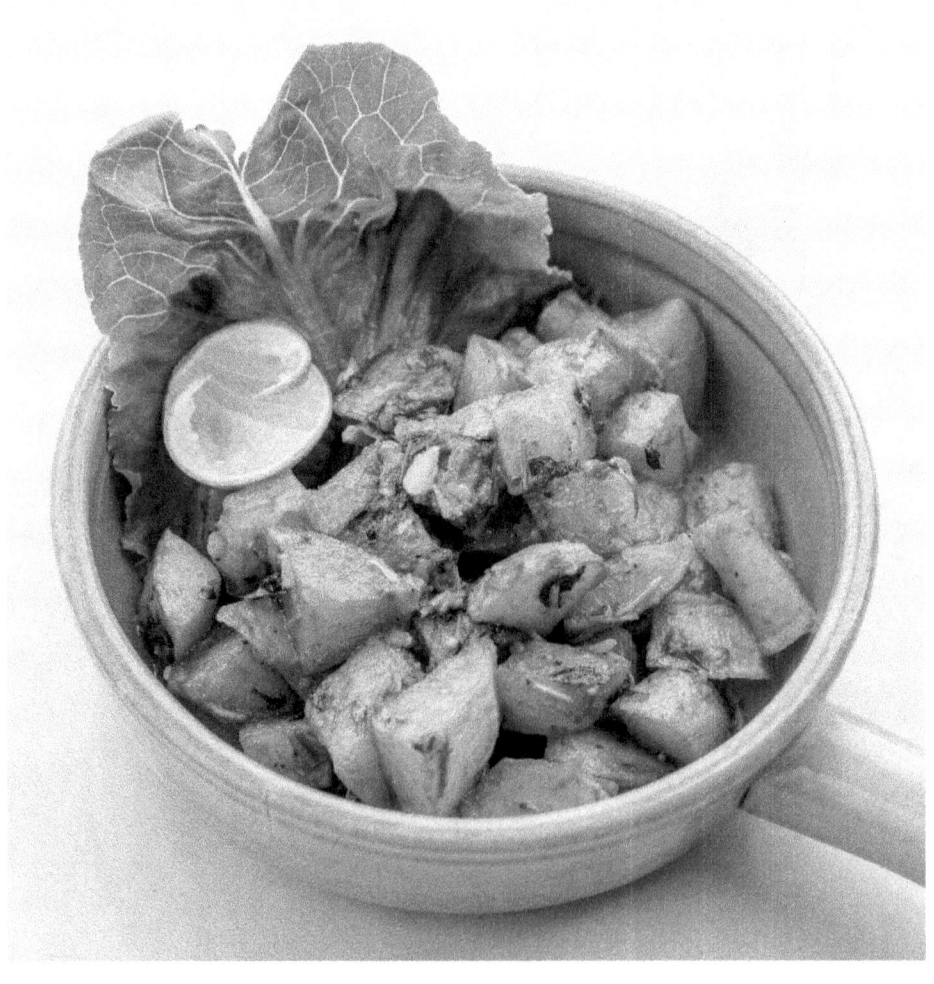

Orange Couscous

Servings: 2

Cooking Time: 15 Minutes

Ingredients:
- 1/3 cup couscous
- ¼ cup of water
- 4 tablespoons orange juice
- ¼ orange, chopped
- 1 teaspoon Italian seasonings
- 1/3 teaspoon salt
- ½ teaspoon butter

Directions:
1. Pour water and orange juice in the pan.
2. Add orange, Italian seasoning, and salt.
3. Bring the liquid to boil and remove it from the heat.
4. Add butter and couscous. Stir well and close the lid.
5. Leave the couscous rest for 10 minutes.

Nutrition Info:Per Serving:calories 149, fat 1.9, fiber 2.1, carbs 28.5, protein 4.1

Walnuts Cucumber Mix

Servings: 2

Cooking Time: 0 Minutes

Ingredients:
- 2 cucumbers, chopped
- 1 tablespoon olive oil
- Salt and black pepper to the taste
- 1 red chili pepper, dried
- 1 tablespoon lemon juice
- 3 tablespoons walnuts, chopped
- 1 tablespoon balsamic vinegar
- 1 teaspoon chives, chopped

Directions:

1. In a bowl, mix the cucumbers with the oil and the rest of the ingredients, toss and serve as a side dish.

Nutrition Info: calories 121, fat 2.3, fiber 2.0, carbs 6.7, protein 2.4

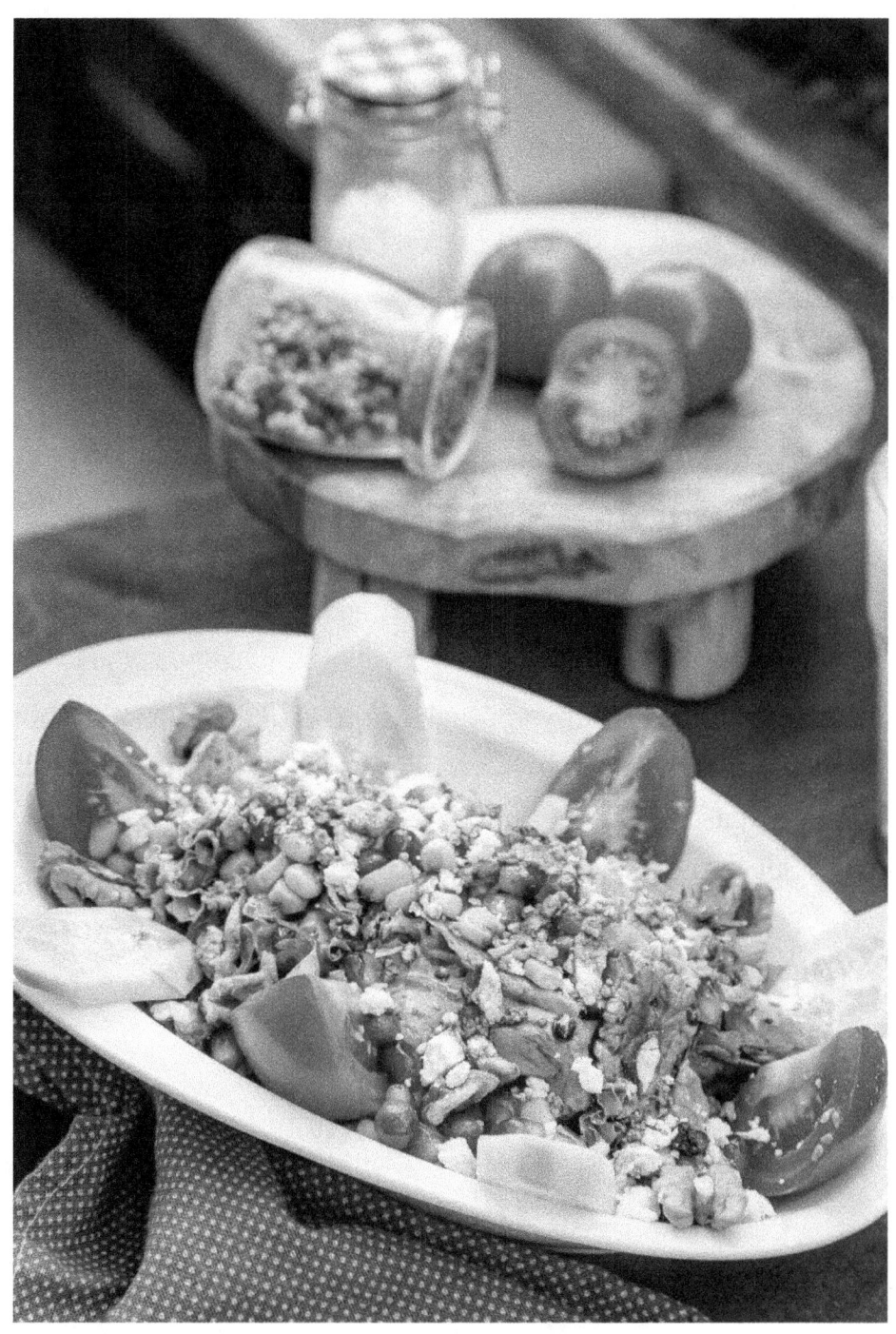

Red Beet Spinach Salad

Servings: 4

Cooking Time: 20 Minutes

Ingredients:
- 3 cups baby spinach
- 2 red beets, cooked and diced
- 1 tablespoon prepared horseradish
- 1 tablespoon apple cider vinegar
- ¼ cup Greek yogurt
- Salt and pepper to taste

Directions:
1. Combine the baby spinach and red beets in a salad bowl.
2. Add the horseradish, vinegar and yogurt and mix well then season with salt and pepper.
3. Serve the salad as fresh as possible.

Nutrition Info: Per Serving:Calories:64 Fat:1.2g Protein:6.4g Carbohydrates:7.5g

Broccoli Spaghetti

Servings: 2

Cooking Time: 10 Minutes

Ingredients:
- 1/3 cup broccoli
- 7 oz whole grain spaghetti
- 2 oz Parmesan, shaved
- ½ teaspoon ground black pepper
- 1 cup water, for cooking

Directions:
1. Chop the broccoli into the small florets.
2. Pour water in the pan. Bring it to boil.
3. Add broccoli florets and spaghetti.
4. Close the lid and cook the ingredients for 10 minutes.
5. Then drain water.
6. Add ground black pepper and shaved Parmesan. Shake the spaghetti well.

Nutrition Info:Per Serving:calories 430, fat 8.8, fiber 9.3, carbs 72.4, protein 23.6

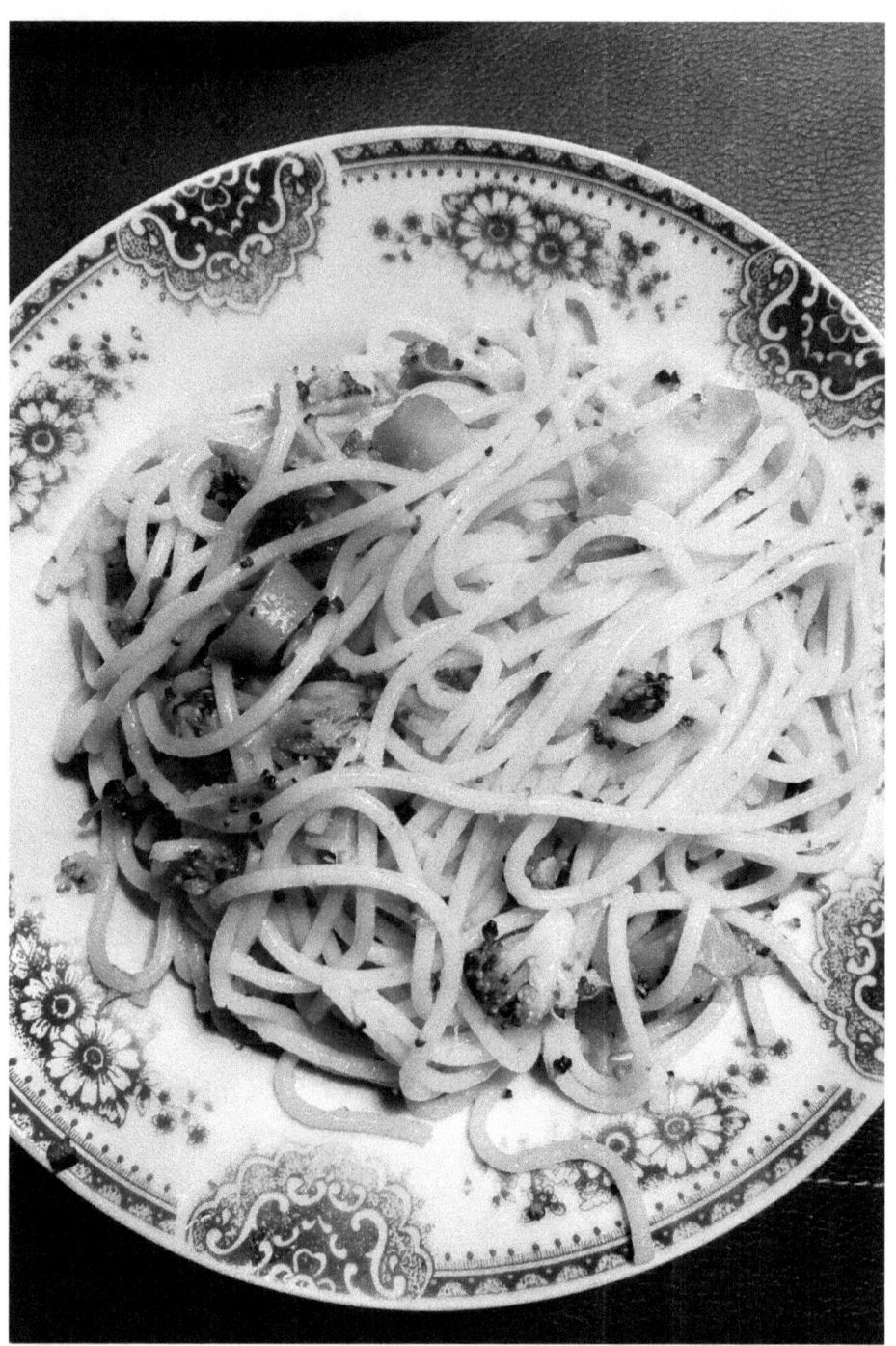

Leeks Sauté

Servings: 4

Cooking Time: 15 Minutes

Ingredients:
- 2 pounds leeks, sliced
- 2 tablespoons chicken stock
- 2 tablespoons tomato paste
- 1 tablespoon olive oil
- 2 tablespoons thyme, chopped
- Salt and black pepper to the taste

Directions:

1. Heat up a pan with the oil over medium heat, add the leeks and brown for 5 minutes.
2. Add the rest of the ingredients, toss, increase the heat to medium-high and cook for 10 minutes more.
3. Divide everything between plates and serve as a side dish.

Nutrition Info: calories 200, fat 11.4, fiber 5.6, carbs 16.4, protein 3.6

Whole-wheat Soft Dinner Dough And Rolls

Servings: 5
Cooking Time: 20-25 Minutes

Ingredients:
- 2 tablespoons yeast
- 1/2 cup warm
- 1/2 cup softened butter
- 1/4 cup honey
- 3 eggs
- 1 cup warm buttermilk (or milk)
- 4 1/2 cups whole-wheat flour
- 1 1/2 teaspoons salt

Directions:
1. Dissolve the yeast in the warm water in a bowl or a glass measuring cup, stirring with a whisk, then set aside.
2. In the bowl of a stand mixer, put the softened butter. Add the honey; cream together using the paddle attachment.
3. Add the eggs; beat, scraping the butter from the bowl sides. Add the warm buttermilk and then the yeast mixture. The mixture will not be smooth and you'll see butter lumps floating. Add the whole-wheat flour and the salt; mix well.

4. Change to the dough hook; knead for a couple of minutes. You just need to lose the extreme stickiness of the dough, but not to develop the gluten. If needed, add a couple of tablespoons of flour. To test, touch the dough surface with a finger. No dough should stick on your finger even though it will look sticky. The dough should still be sticking to the bowl, but should not stick on our finger.

5. When you achieved the correct texture, cover the bowl with towel, and let sit for 1 hour at room temperature. The dough will rise, but it will not double.

6. Transfer the dough onto a floured surface. Knead with your hands a few times, cover with a towel, and let rest for 3 minutes.

7. Meanwhile, generously butter the sides and the bottom of a 9x13-inch pan.

8. Flatten it into an even rectangle shape, roughly about the size of the pan. With a knife, cut the dough into 24 pieces.

9. Now shape them into dinner rolls. If you are right-handed, form your left hand into a circle, the tipoff the thumb almost touching the pointing the middle finger. With your right hand, take a dough and push it up through the hand circle, forming the rounded top. Now turn the ball over and pinch the ends to come together. With the round side up, place the seam side down in the prepared dish - six balls down and fur balls across. The doughs should be touching the pan. Cover with the towel and let rise for 1 more hour. Set a timer for 45 minutes. Start preheating the

oven to 350F during the last 15 minutes of letting the dough rise. After 1 hour, the dough will rise and they will be touching each other.

10. Bake for about 20 to 25 minutes or until golden brown. Rotate the pan 180 degrees for an even browning. As soon as they come out from the oven, brush thee tops with softened butter. As soon as they are cooled to warm, pull the rolls out of the pan and pull them apart to serve.

Nutrition Info:Per Serving:135 cal., 4.7 g fat (2.7 g sat. fat), 32 mg chol., 194 mg sodium, 68 mg pot., 19.7 total carb., 0.8 fiber, 3.5 g sugar, and 3.6 g protein.

Peppers And Lentils Salad

Servings: 4

Cooking Time: 0 Minutes

Ingredients:
- 14 ounces canned lentils, drained and rinsed
- 2 spring onions, chopped
- 1 red bell pepper, chopped
- 1 green bell pepper, chopped
- 1 tablespoon fresh lime juice
- 1/3 cup coriander, chopped
- 2 teaspoon balsamic vinegar

Directions:

1. In a salad bowl, combine the lentils with the onions, bell peppers and the rest of the ingredients, toss and serve.

Nutrition Info: calories 200, fat 2.45, fiber 6.7, carbs 10.5, protein 5.6

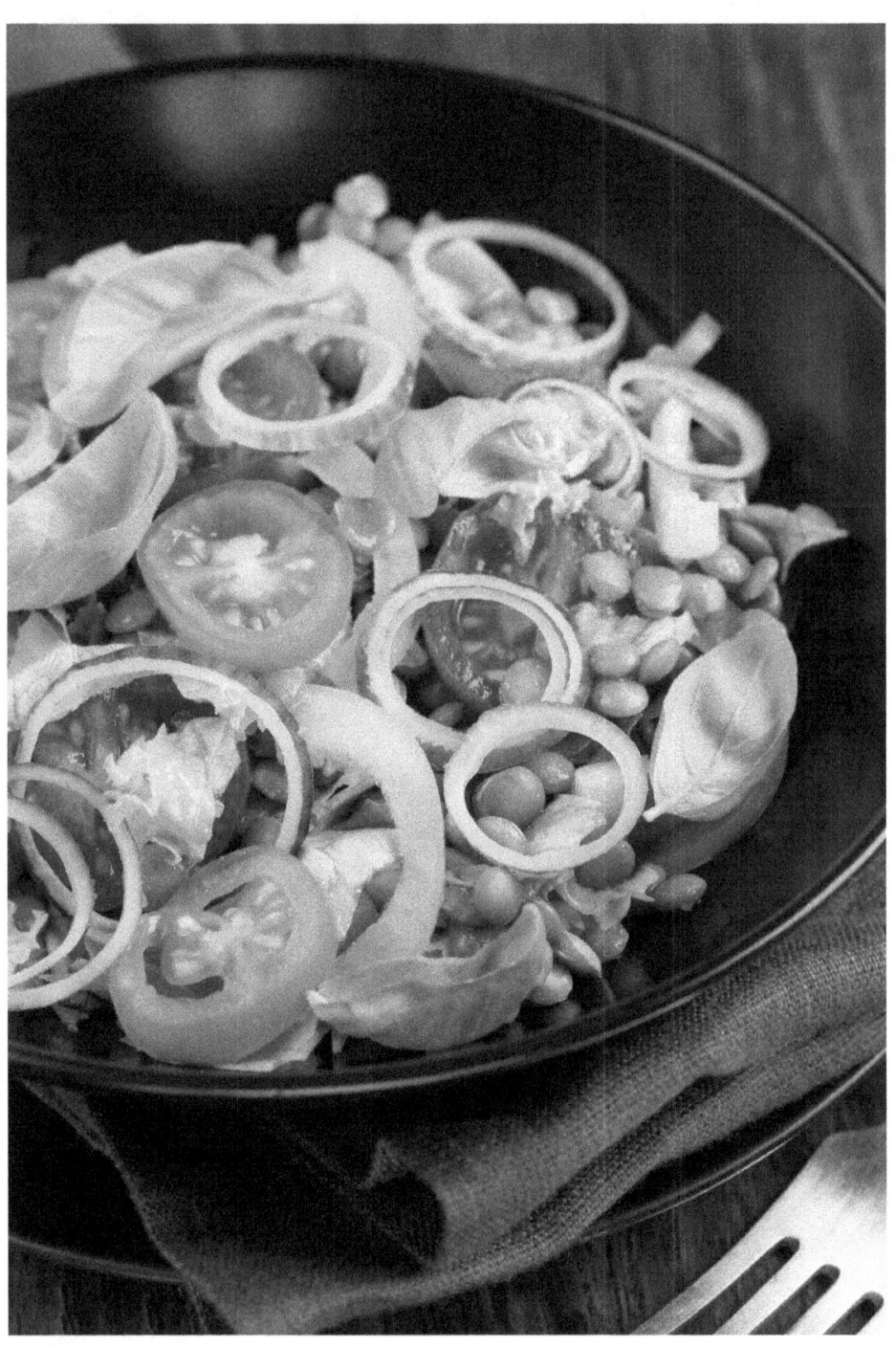

www.ingramcontent.com/pod-product-compliance
Lightning Source LLC
Chambersburg PA
CBHW070722030426
42336CB00013B/1891